BEYOND OBAMACARE

BEYOND OBAMACARE

LIFE, DEATH, AND SOCIAL POLICY

JAMES S. HOUSE

Russell Sage Foundation • New York

The Russell Sage Foundation

The Russell Sage Foundation, one of the oldest of America's general purpose foundations, was established in 1907 by Mrs. Margaret Olivia Sage for "the improvement of social and living conditions in the United States." The Foundation seeks to fulfill this mandate by fostering the development and dissemination of knowledge about the country's political, social, and economic problems. While the Foundation endeavors to assure the accuracy and objectivity of each book it publishes, the conclusions and interpretations in Russell Sage Foundation publications are those of the authors and not of the Foundation, its Trustees, or its staff. Publication by Russell Sage, therefore, does not imply Foundation endorsement.

Library of Congress Cataloging-in-Publication Data

House, James S., 1944– , author.
Beyond Obamacare : life, death, and social policy / James S. House.
p. ; cm.
Includes bibliographical references and index.
ISBN 978-0-87154-477-3 (pbk. : alk. paper) — ISBN 978-1-61044-849-9 (ebook)
I. Russell Sage Foundation, issuing body. II. Title.
[DNLM: 1. Health Care Reform—economics—United States. 2. Health Services Accessibility—economics—United States. 3. Health Status Disparities—United States. 4. Socioeconomic Factors—United States. WA 540 AA1]
RA445
326.10973—dc23 2014045744

The paper used in this publication meets the minimum requirements of American National Standard for Information Sciences—Permanence of Paper for Printed Library Materials. ANSI Z39.48-1992.

Text design by Suzanne Nichols

RUSSELL SAGE FOUNDATION
112 East 64th Street, New York, New York 10065
10 9 8 7 6 5 4 3 2 1

This book is dedicated to

Wendy Fisher House

The love of my life and partner in the social science of health

And our children

Jeffrey Taylor House and Erin Heather House

Who have contributed so much to our fortunate conditions of life

And to two colleagues

Robert L. "Bob" Kahn

Whose pioneering work on social determinants of health and almost four decades of colleagueship have stimulated and supported all the work culminating in this book

And Robert F. "Bob" Schoeni

Who, through his remarkable gift for interdisciplinary collaboration in research and writing, has led me and others to understand more deeply the relations of social science and policy to health science and policy

Contents

List of Illustrations

About the Author

James S. House is Angus Campbell Distinguished University Professor Emeritus of Survey Research, Public Policy, and Sociology at the University of Michigan.

Preface

THIS BOOK seeks to move American health policy "Beyond Obamacare" in two senses. First, for many reasons we need to get beyond the continuing political conflict over whether we should or should not have Obamacare. The Patient Protection and Affordable Care Act (ACA) has been legislated, it has passed Supreme Court review, and it is being implemented with increasing effectiveness in both "red" and "blue" states. It addresses a critical need of American health policy—to make health insurance coverage as universal as possible, both for the good of those in need of health care who have heretofore lacked insurance and for the good of public and private insurance systems, which become more cost-effective as coverage becomes more universal. There are undoubtedly many ways in which we can improve both the existing legislation and its implementation. Refining and improving the Affordable Care Act is a worthy, hopefully bipartisan, endeavor that will require getting beyond the expensive and essentially fruitless revisiting of whether Obamacare should be the established and advancing law of the land that it is.

Ultimately, and much more important, we must get beyond the view of Obamacare as all that we can or should do to deal with the serious health policy problems of our nation. Seeing our health policy problem as mainly one of increasing insurance coverage and making our health care system more cost-effective (as American health policy currently does and has largely done for decades) is to miss the essential, and truly paradoxical, nature of the serious health policy crisis in which we are ever more deeply enmeshed and which is increasingly exceptional among all similarly developed or wealthy nations. America's lack of a system of universal health insurance or health care system remains quite exceptional among economically developed nations. But even more exceptional is the paradox that even as we continue to spend more for health care and insurance than any other nation, our levels of population health have only worsened relative to all comparably economically developed nations and are now worsening even absolutely for some portions of the American population and on some health indicators for the entire population.

The first goal of this book is to clearly delineate this paradoxical crisis (chapter 1) and to show why America's solely supply-side approach to health—seeking to provide more and better health care and insurance to more and more people (Obamacare being the latest example)—has not, will not, and cannot resolve our paradoxical crisis of spending more and more on health care and insurance yet getting less and less in terms of health (chapter 2). At the margins, the ACA may slightly moderate the growth of health spending or slightly improve population health parameters, though even that remains to be seen. But like any supply-side health policy or reform, it is incapable of substantially ameliorating America's increasingly high levels of health spending and worsening population health outcomes.

To simultaneously make substantial reductions in spending while reversing the worsening of America's population health requires a focus on a demand-side health policy, one that will make the population healthier, largely by non-biomedical means, so as to reduce the need and demand for health care and hence expenditures for health care and insurance. Chapter 3 explores why we are so fixated on health care and insurance as the sole objects of health policy when, in fact, the major determinants of health lie *not* in medical care but rather in the conditions of life and work, especially changes in those conditions at the level of populations.

Conditions of life and work are highly variable across the population, yet they are largely determined by a few fundamental factors—socioeconomic position, race-ethnicity, and gender—that structure individuals' experience of and exposure to virtually all of the major risk factors for health. Thus, some people have highly favorable profiles of health and the risk factors for health, while others have highly negative ones. When we couple these factors with the biological limits on health and longevity (chapters 4 and 5), we see that the major need and opportunity for improving population health—and thereby reducing health spending—lies in improving not only the health but the conditions of life and work of those in the lower socioeconomic half of our population. Because more and more of those with the best levels of health and conditions of life are able to approach the biological limits of human health, the potential gains from providing this advantaged population, including its older members, with more medical care or improving their conditions of life and work are much more marginal.

As chapter 6 shows, we actually know a great deal about how and why demand-side health policy is generally more powerful, and certainly more cost-effective, in improving health and hence reducing health spending. And we know more all the time about the causal impacts of major areas of public (and private) policy, especially social policy, on health in ways that are at least equally as cost-effective as health care, and generally more so (chapter 7). And contrary to what we might expect, healthier individuals and populations actually spend less on health care (chapter 8).

Thus, we do not get healthy by spending more and more for health care, but rather by spending more and doing more to create healthful conditions of life and work (chapter 9). This must be the centerpiece of a more demand-side health policy going forward. Such a policy would pay increased attention to the health effects of a range of "nonhealth" policies, especially those that affect the fundamental causes of conditions of life and work—socioeconomic position and other socially constructed attributes associated with race-ethnicity and gender, such as segregation and discrimination.

This is a book about health science and health policy. It is also a book about social science and social policy. Most of all, it is a book about the relationships of social science and policy to health science and policy, and vice versa. It will have succeeded at one level if it more clearly delineates the paradox of America's growing crisis of health care and health—spending more and more on health care and insurance, yet getting less and less in terms of health. It will have succeeded at another level if it demonstrates how and why supply-side approaches to health policy and reforms—all fixated on getting more and better health care to more and more people—have not, will not, and cannot more than marginally improve the two key components of America's growing paradoxical crisis of health care and health. At best, these supply-side approaches can have only slight impacts on restraining the growth of health expenditures or improving America's population health parameters. This book will have succeeded at an even more fundamental level if it not only overturns the conventional wisdom that health care is the major determinant of health but also creates a new understanding that health is a function of the conditions of life and work that we experience day in and day out as individuals and as a society.

And *Beyond Obamacare* will have succeeded most completely if it has a hand in redirecting health policy to focus more on the broad range of nonhealth policies—especially those involving socioeconomic position, race-ethnicity, or gender—that shape the conditions of life and work, especially among the half or so of our population who live and work in disadvantaged conditions and whose health is consequently affected. And conversely, this book will have succeeded if it affects the formulation and evolution of nonhealth policies to account for their often unrecognized health effects as well as the non-health-related ends to which they are more explicitly directed.

Thus, in the end, the nature and quality of our health and health policy depend on the nature and quality of our broader societal policies, practices, and conditions of life and work, both public and private. The sooner and more completely we recognize and act on the basis of this fundamental insight, the sooner and more completely we will be able to resolve our paradoxical crisis of health care and health. Doing so will also contribute to alleviating many of the other fiscal, social, and political crises that confront our nation domestically and enable us to better deal with the challenges of an increasingly global world.

None of the chapters of this book is highly novel; all of their content is considered in more depth elsewhere. What is new and valuable in *Beyond Obamacare* is what the pioneering epidemiologist John Snow termed the "orderly arrangement [of established facts] into chains of inference which extend beyond the bounds of direct observation."[1]

Acknowledgments

As THE dedication suggests, this book is the result and culmination of my life and career to date and hence reflects debts to many who have stimulated, helped, and supported me along the way. My parents, James House Jr. and Virginia Sturgis House, to whom I dedicated my first and only other sole-authored book about thirty years ago, instilled in me a curiosity and love of learning about the world and supported me in all I did as long as they lived. Halsey G. House was a model big brother when we were growing up and has now given thorough and thoughtful commentary on the first publisher's draft of this book from the perspective of a research engineer and creative and committed teacher of science. I have also been fortunate to have studied in three educational institutions that fostered a broad, interdisciplinary perspective on general education, the study of social life, and their application to the public interest: the public schools of Springfield (Delaware County), Pennsylvania, Haverford College, and the University of Michigan (UM).

Excellent as they were, none of these educational institutions offered any formal coursework on the relations between social science and health, much less social policy and health. I was fortunate during my graduate work at UM, however, to stumble on the impact of stress on health while searching for a better theoretical approach to understanding how, when, and why social stresses and strains give rise to various social attitudes and individual and collective actions. My still-senior colleague Robert L. Kahn and several others—Sidney Cobb, John R. P. French, and Stanislav Kasl—had developed one of the first research programs on the social environment and health, and I did my dissertation in social psychology with them, studying occupational stress and health in the Tecumseh Community Health Study of the UM School of Public Health.

Yet another fortuitous turn landed me in my first academic job in the Sociology Department of Duke University, with connections to Duke's Center for the Study of Aging and Human Development and the Department of Epidemiology in the School of Public Health at the University of North Carolina at Chapel Hill (UNC). All of these units also happened to be pioneers in documenting the relations of psychosocial factors to health. To my mentors at Michigan were added Kurt Back, Alan Kerckhoff, Redford Williams, and especially George Maddox at Duke; and at UNC, Bertram Kaplan, Anthony McMichael, Sherman James, and especially, though from a distance, John Cassel, one of the pioneers of social epidemiology. Cobb at UM and Cassel at UNC both stimulated and supported my work on occupational stress and health and led me and others into the study of social relationships and health, which became the focus of my research for over a decade that spanned the end of my time in the Research Triangle in 1978 and the beginning of the more than thirty-six years I have now been a faculty member and research scientist back at Michigan—yet another serendipitous transition little foreseen before it was upon me.

As I try to convey to potential recruits, UM and Ann Arbor are wonderfully stimulating and supportive places to work and live. Central to this supportive environment is UM's extraordinary culture of interdisciplinary education and research, embodied in the Survey Research Center (SRC) and Institute for Social Research (ISR), which have provided my intellectual and research home during my entire UM career. While the Department of Sociology has been my principal academic and disciplinary home, first the School of Public Health (especially its Departments of Epidemiology, Biostatistics, and Health Behavior and Education) and over the last decade the Ford School of Public Policy have welcomed me as a colleague and collaborator in work that initially focused on social determinants and disparities in health and, more recently, their relations to health policy and broader public policy. Leaders of all of these units have been invariably welcoming and supportive, especially F. Thomas Juster and Howard Schumann, directors of ISR and SRC, respectively, and Angus Campbell, the emeritus director of both; Bill Gamson, Reynolds Farley, and Mayer Zald, chairs of the Department of Sociology; Victor Hawthorne, chair of the Epidemiology Department; and Rebecca Blank and Susan Collins, successive deans of the Ford School.

From the end of my time at Duke and UNC through the present, my research and predoctoral and postdoctoral training have been substantially and continuously supported by key external funders. Most significant and continuous has been the support of the National Institutes of Health (NIH), first through the National Institute of Mental Health and the National Heart, Lung, and Blood Institute, and for over three decades through the National Institute on Aging. For just over two decades, the Robert Wood Johnson Foundation (RWJF) has also been a major source of financial and social support through three programs that have represented important stimuli and supports for research on social determinants and disparities in health and their applications to health policy—the RWJF Health Policy Scholars Program, the RWJF Investigators in Health Policy Program, and the RWJF Health and Society Scholars Program. At a time when I believe the relevance of work on social determinants and disparities in health to health policy and broader social policy has never been greater—and is becoming more so with each passing day—I hope that RWJF's support for this important work is not diminished but rather strengthened by its termination of these and other RWJF human capital programs to pursue a new, but still evolving initiative for a "Culture of Health." Likewise, in a time of tight budgeting, I hope that NIH will expand rather than shrink its support for research on the impact of social factors and social policy on health and health policy.

Two wonderful sabbaticals were responsible for the genesis of the ideas for this book. The first was in 2005–2006 at the Center for Advanced Study in the Social and Behavioral Sciences, then directed by Claude Steele. The volume was written and completed through the Russell Sage Foundation (RSF), beginning while I was at RSF in 2010–2011 with the drafting of the first half, with the support of then-president Eric Wanner, and continuing to its completion and publication under RSF's new president, and my colleague, Sheldon Danziger. RSF's director of publications, Suzanne Nichols, has been a steady source of judiciously mixed inspiration, support, and goading, for all of which I will be forever grateful. Claire Gabriel, RSF's director of information services, and Galo Falchettore, a research computer specialist, provided invaluable research and graphic support while I was at RSF and collaborated with Robert Melendez of our staff, whose computing expertise has been a godsend with final graphic and reference updates.

Finally, I have been blessed to collaborate with and learn from many people in the preparation of this book and all that led up to it. In acknowledging some, even many, I necessarily leave many unmentioned, but not unappreciated. Among those as yet not mentioned and who have been major collaborators in research and training, though with no direct role in the particular synthesis of this book, are: Jennifer Ailshire, Jenny Brand, Sarah Burgard, Philippa Clarke, Ana Diez Roux, Michael Elliott, Pamela Herd, Regula Herzog, Maggie Hicken, Barbara Israel, James Jackson, Graham Kalton, George Kaplan, Ronald Kessler, Karl Landis, Paula Lantz, Hedy Lee, James Lepkowski, John Lynch, Neil Mehta, Helen Metzner, Paul Mohai, Jim Morgan, Jeffrey Morenoff, Marc Musick, Steve Raudenbush, Cynthia Robbins, Debra Umberson, David Williams, and Camille Wortman. I have been blessed with talented and committed professional and clerical support staff without whom our research and training program and the publications and data sets emanating from them would not be possible: Cathy Doherty, Debbie Fitch, Mary Jo Griewahn, Marie Klatt, Robin Lounsbury, Robert Melendez, Rich Mero, Sue Meyer, and Barb Strane. Cathy Doherty's role in the preparation of this book has been extraordinary. Without her careful and thoughtful handling of all aspects of the preparation of the entire volume, it either would never have come to pass or would have contained many errors of omission and commission from which she saved me and the book. Rick Price has been a long-term colleague and thoughtful commenter on this book.

I have benefited greatly from the careful and thoughtful reading of the publisher's draft by two reviewers chosen by RSF, one of whom identified himself: not only in this review but in many other ways over my career, David Mechanic has been a source of great support and insightful feedback. Many others have responded generously, thoughtfully, and constructively to my requests for their comments. Beyond those already noted, these include: David Fisher, Joel Howell, James Knickman, John Mullahy, Stephanie Robert, Pamela Russo, Jason Schnittker, Nancy and Roger Smith, and Laura Wherry.

A number of colleagues have gone beyond the call of duty in providing comments that were exceptionally encouraging and motivating and/or detailed and instructive. Two of my colleagues in the sociology of health, Renee Anspach and Mark Chesler, provided quite detailed, thoughtful, and constructive commentaries and edits, especially from the perspective of great appreciation for and knowledge of the health care and insurance system. Sherman James, my admired colleague at both Duke/UNC and UM, came through with his usual combination of generous support and incisive rigor regarding the entire manuscript, within a very narrow corridor in his always busy schedule. David Kindig, one of the pioneers and still leaders in science and policy regarding population health, was once again the cogent and supportive colleague he has always been. Alvin Tarlov, another iconic leader and longtime supportive colleague and mentor in the field of social medicine and population health, provided his usual thoughtful and upbeat input at a point when the revision process might otherwise have lagged. My longest-term senior colleague, Bob Kahn, at age ninety-six, was a judicious source of encouragement and constructive critique, adding once again to all he has done to stimulate and support my work since early in my graduate career; he is certainly worthy of inclusion among those to whom this book is dedicated. Finally, Bob Schoeni provided his always judicious, constructive, and forward-looking input at several points in the development of the manuscript. It was my work with him on our edited volume (with George Kaplan and Harold Pollack), *Making Americans Healthier* (2008), that solidified and edified my growing interest in the relation of research on social determinants and health to both health policy and broader social policy. If a major health problem had not so unfairly intervened in his life, we might have collaborated again on this book. His inclusion among those to whom the book is dedicated reflects my appreciation of what he has done for me, and for so many others, to foster a broad, interdisciplinary, and policy-oriented approach to research and writing on social determinants and disparities in health.

The credit for any degree to which this book reaches a readership beyond researchers and students of social determinants and disparities in health—as I hope that it will—goes to my other beloved nonagenarian friend, Rhea Kish, whose editorial skills and work are reflected in virtually every page—indeed, every paragraph and sentence—of this book. That Rhea has chosen to make my book perhaps the last of her major editorial accomplishments is both deeply appreciated and touching. The book is much better in substance and style as a result of her magnificent and magnanimous effort. Cynthia Buck's thoughtful, careful, and considerate copyediting has furthered the process that Rhea began. Bytheway Publishing Services has ably, efficiently, and collaboratively converted the jumble of an edited manuscript into its present form.

Finally, Wendy Fisher House has both read and encouraged this work from its inception, perhaps most importantly in her efforts to make sure that it did not move as slowly as most things that I do. And our life together has always been a source of inspiration. Jeff and Erin are too busy doing well and good in their own lives to read their father's turgid drafts, but they too have been a source of inspiration. Individually and together, I hope and believe that Wendy, Jeff, Erin, and I have created conditions of life and work that have been healthful for us and others. Certainly my family has done this for me, and constitute the real meaning of life.

All of these contributors have only made this work and my fortunate life better and are in no way responsible for any remaining problems in this book.

Chapter 1

Health, Health Care, and Health Policy in America: A Contradiction Wrapped in a Paradox Inside an Enigma

IN 2009 and 2010, the United States engaged in its most intensive debate over health policy in almost two decades. The outcome was the most comprehensive health care and insurance legislation in half a century—the Patient Protection and Affordable Care Act (PPACA or just ACA, aka Obamacare), which remains a central political and policy issue. In varying ways and to different degrees, all of the actors in this process have been motivated by two seemingly contradictory goals. The first is to reduce, or at least slow the growth of, increasingly burdensome costs and expenditures for health care and insurance—costs borne by individuals, families, businesses, and government at all levels, and thus by American society as a whole. The second goal is to enhance the accessibility and quality of health care for all Americans, not only as a matter of social justice but also because universal coverage generally improves the cost-effectiveness of any insurance system. It remains unclear, however, whether we can simultaneously reduce or limit health spending, while also enhancing the quality and accessibility of health care and improving the health of all Americans. In theory, these two goals are contradictory, as they may also be in fact, at least within the confines of current policy discussion and directions.

Underlying this putative *contradiction* is a *paradox*: while it is uncertain whether and how we can improve health for all Americans by spending less for health care, it is even more questionable whether spending more for health care and insurance, or even improving its quality, can commensurately improve the actual health of the American population. Indeed, the United States is in the grips of what I term a "paradoxical crisis" of health care and health: we spend more and more for health care and insurance, both absolutely and relative to all other nations in the world, yet we get less and less in terms of improved health, as shown in major indicators of population health.

America's Paradoxical Crisis of Health Care and Health

Over the past half-century, U.S. spending on health care has outstripped health spending by every country in the world. Yet our standing on a number of indicators of population health—such as life expectancy, infant mortality, and, more recently, maternal mortality—has been declining from among the best in the world in the 1950s to worse today than virtually every developed nation in the world, as well as a number of developing ones. We are even beginning to see some evidence of *absolute declines* in the health of portions of the American population. Such declines have not been seen anywhere in recent decades except in the face of major epidemics (such as AIDS in Africa), wars, natural disasters, or massive political and economic transformations (such as from communism to market economies in Eastern Europe). How the wealthiest and most powerful nation in the world, and also by far the greatest spender on health care and insurance, could experience declining relative and perhaps even absolute levels of population health constitutes a very profound paradox.

At this point, both the rise in spending for health and the relative, and absolute for some, declines in population health seem likely to continue for as long as we can reasonably project or predict. As figure 1.1 shows, over the last half-century U.S. (the heavy solid line in figs. 1.1 to 1.5, 1.7, and 1.8) spending on health and health care as a percentage of gross domestic product (GDP) has moved from close to, but not at, the top of all countries in the world in 1960 to now being 50 percent or more *above* all other comparably developed nations.[1] The 18 percent of GDP we spend today—over three times the level in 1960—is likely to increase both relatively and absolutely to 20 percent or more by the third decade of the twenty-first century.[2] Data on per capita health spending reveal very similar trends.

Another benchmark for current levels of health spending is national defense spending, which has historically constituted the largest single area of government and even GDP expenditures. After World War II, defense spending reached a peak of 15 percent of GDP at the height of the Cold War in 1952, but it has declined since then to the current levels of 5 percent or less of GDP, even while the United States fights multiple wars on foreign soil. What President Dwight Eisenhower termed the

Figure 1.1 GDP Spent on Health in the United States and Four Comparably Wealthy Nations, 1960–2012 (with Projections for the United States from 2013 to 2023)

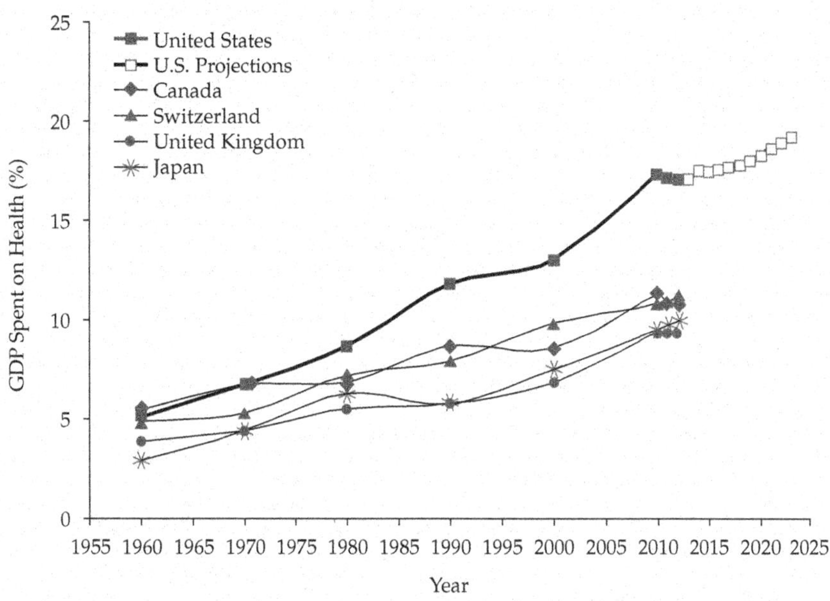

Source: Author compilation based on OECD iLibrary and OECD.StatExtracts (1960—2012); and Centers for Medicare and Medicaid Services, Office of the Actuary (U.S. 2010–2023).

"military-industrial complex" has been superseded by an even larger "medical-biotechnology complex."[3]

If levels of health and gains in health in the United States were in any reasonable way commensurate with our burgeoning expenditures for medical care and insurance, one would expect us to have at least somewhat outstripped all nations in levels of population health. The situation is paradoxically quite to the contrary. Figures 1.2 to 1.5 show the trends in life expectancy both at birth and at age sixty-five for men and women over the same countries and a similar time period as in figure 1.1. With the slight exception of male life expectancy at birth (figure 1.2), in each and every case the United States in 1950 stood at or near the top among these five nations (and among all others as well). Yet by the most recent years for which data are available, the United States ended up below the four comparison nations (and below twenty to forty other nations as well, depending on how broad the comparison group is).[4]

Especially notable and disturbing are the trends for American women,

Figure 1.2 Male Life Expectancy at Birth in the United States and Four Comparably Wealthy Nations, 1950–2011

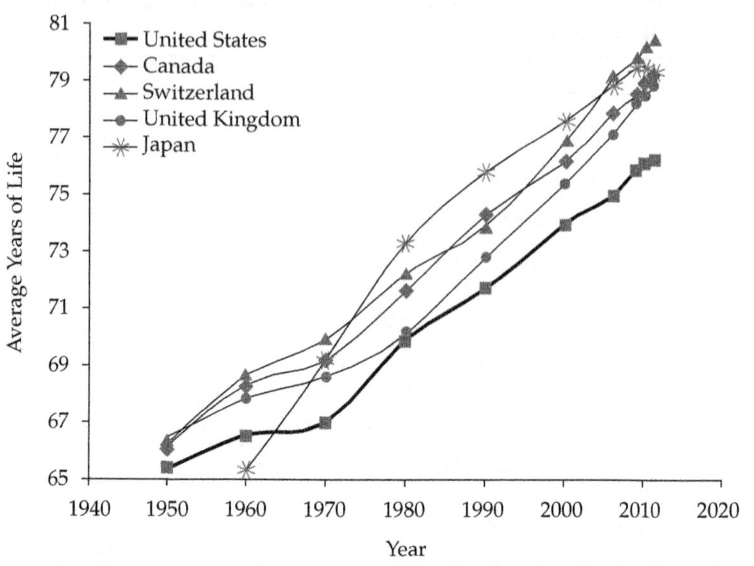

Source: Author compilation based on UN Demographic Yearbook (1950) and OECD.Stat Extracts (1960–2011).

Figure 1.3 Female Life Expectancy at Birth in the United States and Four Comparably Wealthy Nations, 1950–2011

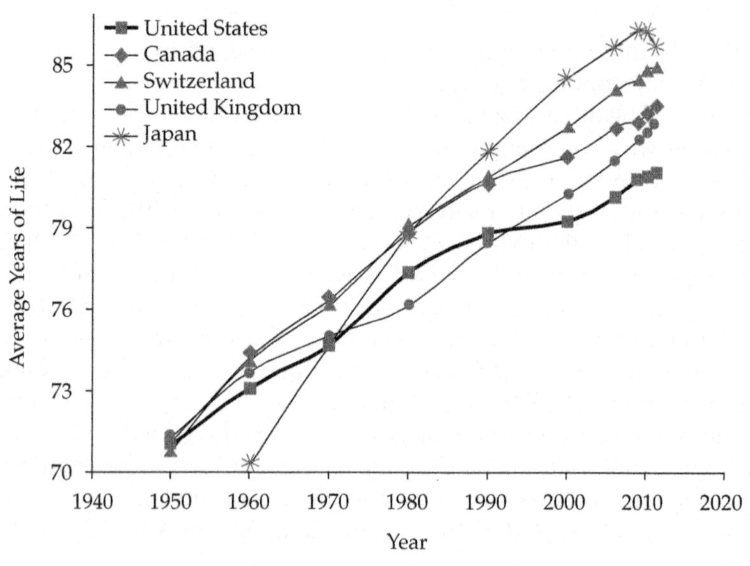

Source: Author compilation based on UN Demographic Yearbook (1950) and OECD.Stat Extracts (1960–2011).

Figure 1.4 Male Life Expectancy at Age Sixty-Five in the United States and Four Comparably Wealthy Nations, 1950–2011

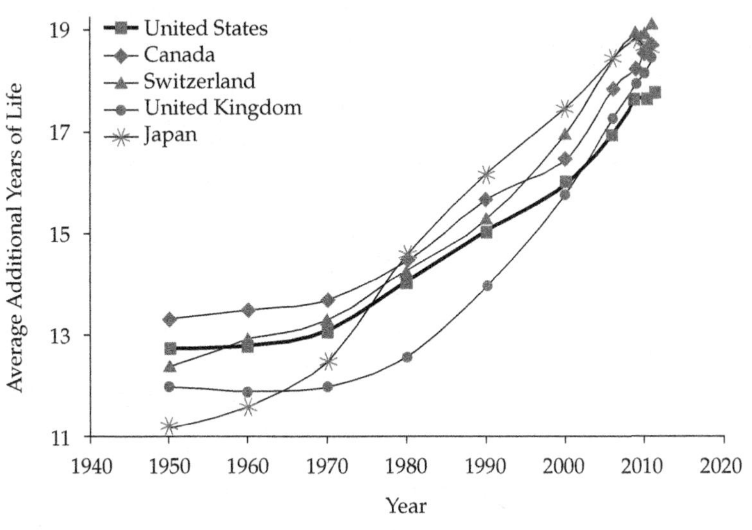

Source: Author compilation based on UN Demographic Yearbook (1950) and OECD.Stat Extracts (1960–2011).

Figure 1.5 Female Life Expectancy at Age Sixty-Five in the United States and Four Comparably Wealthy Nations, 1950–2011

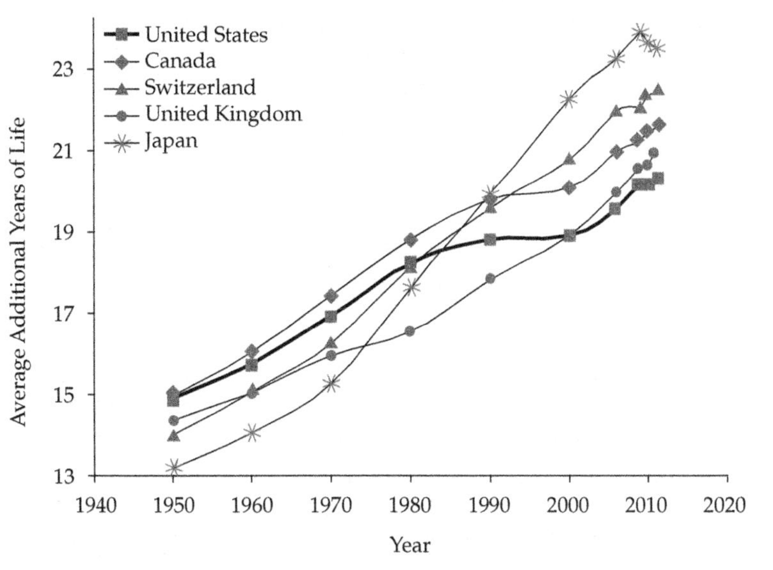

Source: Author compilation based on UN Demographic Yearbook (1950) and OECD.Stat Extracts (1960–2011).

whose life expectancy was at or near the top of the world in the third quarter of the twentieth century. The rate of increase in their life expectancy has slowed dramatically since 1980, and it could *decline absolutely* as the impact of the mid-twentieth-century cigarette smoking epidemic is increasingly felt among women, as it has already been felt among men (women's smoking having both increased and declined later than men's). As can be seen in figures 1.3 and 1.5, since 1950 U.S. women have lost, depending on the age range and country in question, between one and just over six years of life expectancy relative to women in other comparably wealthy nations. Comparing the graphs for men and women, since 1980 women have lost almost three years of the eight-year advantage they had over American men at birth, and almost two and a half years of the four-and-a-half-year advantage they had at age sixty-five. Some geographic areas and population subgroups are even beginning to show absolute declines in female life expectancy.[5]

Figure 1.6 graphically illustrates the absolute declines in life expectancy in portions of the *white* female population, confirming that this is not only, or perhaps even mainly, a problem of disadvantaged minorities. Specifically, figure 1.6 shows that between 1990 and 2008, life expectancy increased steadily by more than three years for white women with sixteen or more years of education (college graduates and above), while gains for women of moderate education (those with either twelve or thirteen to fifteen years of education) were much more moderate (one year or less) over roughly the same period. For white women with less than twelve years of education (those without a high school diploma), life expectancy actually *decreased by five years in less than two decades.*

Figure 1.6 also illustrates the broader problems of social disparities in health that become more central to the argument later in this book, especially in chapters 4 and 5 and continuing in part II. Educational disparities in life expectancy for white women are evident over the entire period from 1990 (and before) to 2008, but grow from being nonmonotonic and at most several years in 1990 to ten years by 2007. Even as the average level of health in the American population is still improving—if at varying rates by gender, socioeconomic position, race-ethnicity, and combinations thereof—educational (and other socioeconomic or racial-ethnic) disparities of ten years or more in life expectancy are more the rule than the exception.

American women's traditional life expectancy advantage over men will continue to shrink, owing to the delayed impact of their increased levels of smoking in the midtwentieth century, and may even disappear, as may have already occurred for black women. Even as the life expectancy gap between American men and women is diminished, however, gains in life expectancy for American men are trailing those of men in

Figure 1.6 Life Expectancy at Birth in the United States, by Years of Education at Age Twenty-Five, for White Females, 1990–2008

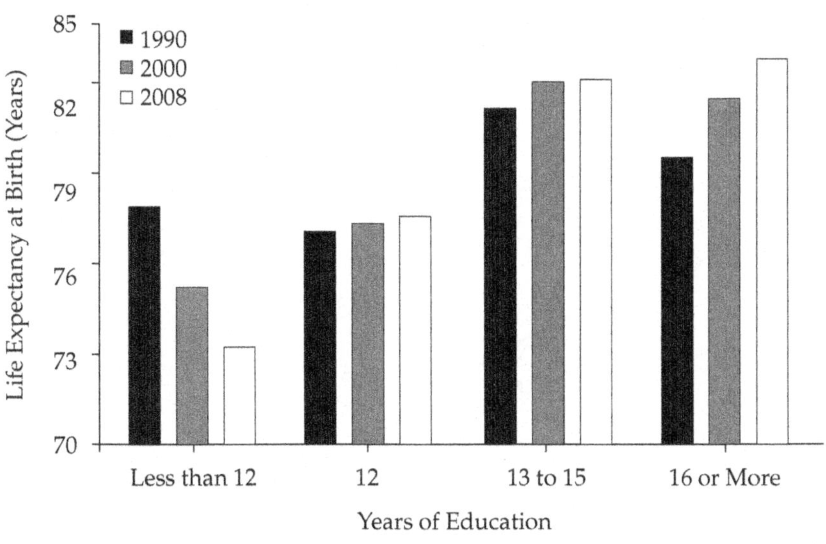

Source: Olshansky et al. (2012, exhibit 2). © 2012 Project HOPE. Reprinted with permission.

other comparably developed countries. We do not yet understand the reasons for all of these changes in life expectancy, but they clearly go beyond smoking and even obesity. If such absolute declines in life expectancy come to characterize a majority and not just a minority of women, and if women's life expectancy decreases to levels at or below men's, it would be unprecedented in a highly developed nation. Previously, such a trend has been seen only in less-developed societies that have severely devalued women and limited their social position and opportunities. Even if absolute overall declines are largely avoided, the relative declines are disturbing enough.

Further evidence of America's relative and even absolute declining levels of population health, both generally and for women, can be seen in figures 1.7 and 1.8, which graph levels of infant and maternal mortality for the same nations and for a similar time period as in figures 1.2 to 1.5 on life expectancy. Declines in infant and maternal mortality played a central role in the almost thirty-year increase in life expectancy in the twentieth century, especially up to 1950. By 1950, the United States had the lowest infant mortality rate (IMR) among the five countries in figure 1.7 (and among all but a handful of others with similarly low rates). Yet today it has the highest IMR compared to these five and more than thirty

Figure 1.7 Infant Mortality in the United States and Four Comparably Wealthy Nations, 1950–2011

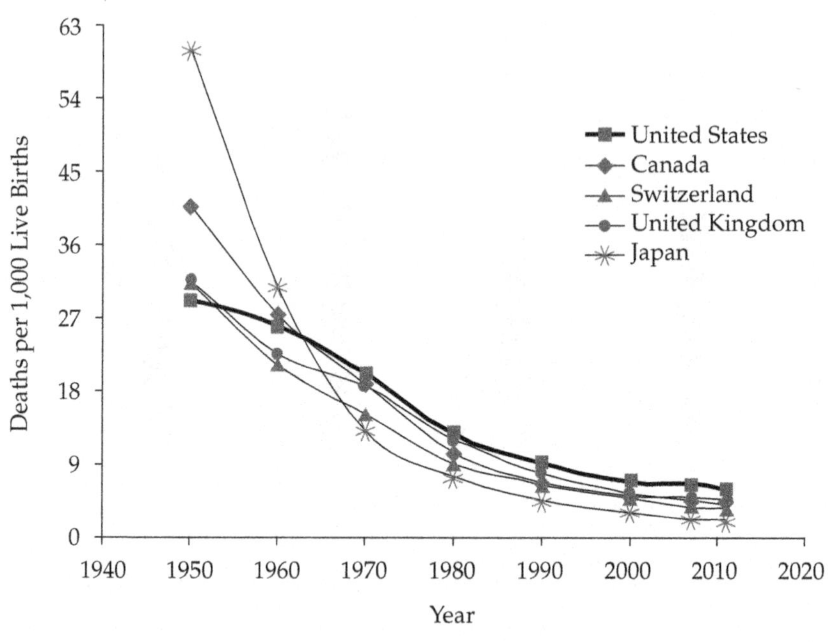

Source: Author compilation based on UN Demographic Yearbook (1950) and OECD.Stat Extracts (1960–2011).

others. Figure 1.8 shows that the U.S. maternal mortality rate in 1970 was also in the lower range of rates among these same five nations (and among all others in the world). Since 1990, maternal mortality has risen steadily, and increasingly sharply, not only relative to all other highly developed countries but also *absolutely* and relative to many less-developed countries. Again, the reasons for this disturbing trend are just beginning to be investigated.

In sum, between 1950 and 1970, the United States was one of the top several nations in the percentage of GDP it spent on health, but we were hardly extraordinary among nations of the Organization for Economic Cooperation and Development (OECD), a consortium that now includes thirty-four of the world's most-developed nations. Since 1970, however, we have become number one in health spending by an increasingly large margin. Paradoxically, America's OECD rankings on many indicators of population health, which were already slipping by 1970, have steadily declined since the 1980s. Today the only OECD nations that consistently rank below the United States on indicators of population health are Mexico, Turkey, Hungary, and the Slovak Republic.

Figure 1.8 Maternal Mortality in the United States and Four Comparably Wealthy Nations, 1970–2010

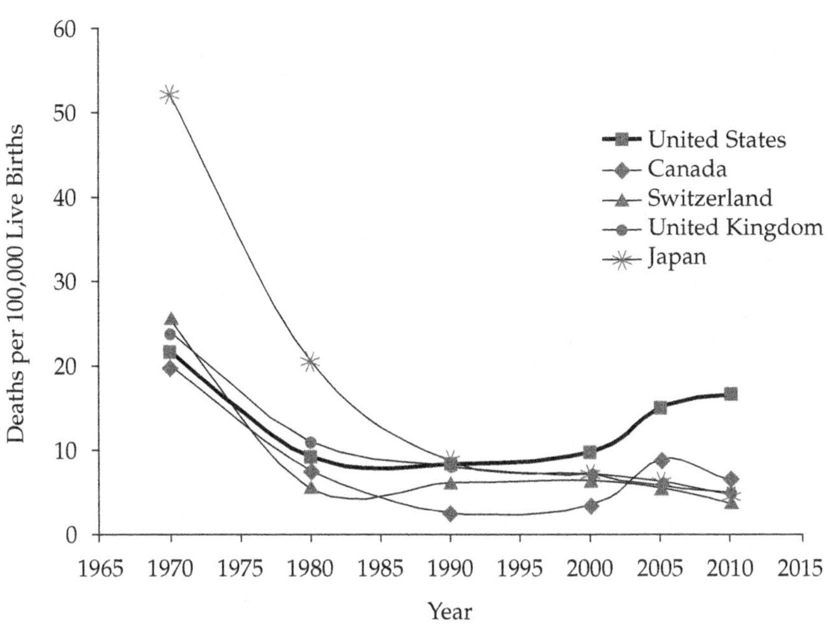

Source: Author compilation based on OECD.StatExtracts (1970–2010) and Centers for Disease Control and Prevention Pregnancy, Mortality Surveillance System (U.S. 2010).

The Enigma: Why and How the Paradoxical Health Crisis Has Arisen

It remains an *enigma* as to why the United States has become mired in this paradoxical crisis of spending more and more on health care and insurance yet getting less and less return in terms of population health. How we can resolve this paradoxical crisis is even more puzzling. Something is woefully wrong with the picture of the United States revealed in figures 1.1 to 1.8, yet we seem incapable of even getting the picture into proper focus, much less making it right. Our understanding of the first element of the paradox, our increased spending, has grown as we have made efforts to, at a minimum, "bend the curve" of growth in health care and insurance spending and perhaps even reduce it. But the central enigma remains unresolved: how do we construct a health policy that dampens the increase in or even reduces spending on health care and insurance while also reversing the clear relative declines—and some absolute declines—in our levels of population health?

Toward a New Health and Health Care Policy in America

While seeking to clarify the enigma of how and why the United States has become so deeply entrenched in its paradoxical crisis of health care and health, this book also suggests how we can resolve the paradox by doing the seemingly contradictory—achieving better population health while reducing health spending. Listening to proponents of health care reform, of almost any type, one might think such a book is not necessary. Have these analysts not already explained how and why America got into this paradoxical crisis, and have they not produced proposals—and in 2010, legislation—that will substantially reduce (or at least slow the growth of) spending for health care while also improving levels of population health? Unfortunately, the answer is decidedly no, for two reasons—one tactical, the other strategic.

Tactically, as we will see in chapter 2, achieving health care reform in the United States has proven exceedingly difficult, even when ultimately somewhat successful, as in 2010. Consequently, any reforms achieved tend to be too little and too late, with little long-term effect on our seemingly inexorable paradox of spending more and more on health care and insurance and getting less and less in terms of population health. Hopefully, the 2010 reforms, if they are not vitiated in the process of being implemented and funded, will provide at least marginally better results. Yet a variety of evidence considered in chapter 2 suggests that even universal access to health care and insurance would only marginally improve population health while probably increasing health spending.

Strategic Reason 1: The Need to Shift from Supply-Side to Demand-Side Policy

We must do all we reasonably can to make this largest sector of our economy as cost-effective as possible. However, to truly rein in spending on health care while also significantly improving population health, we need a totally new strategy. American health policy has increasingly become what economists would call a supply-side policy. That is, the goal is to maintain and improve population health by supplying more and better health care to more and more Americans while trying to manage or reduce the cost of such care. Health care reform—including its latest manifestation—is similarly supply-side reform.

There is almost always a demand-side alternative or complement to supply-side policies, and indeed, successful overall policy is often a mixture of supply-side and demand-side policies. A demand-side health policy would focus on making the population healthier largely by means other than health care and insurance.[6] A healthier population should need, demand, and utilize less—and probably less expensive—health care; thus, expenditures for health care and insurance at all levels of society should be reduced. These savings, in turn, could help to fund critical investments in other areas to improve population health and society more generally.

The relationship between supply-side and demand-side policy can be seen in many other policy areas and problems. In the area of energy and the environment, we seek to ensure supplies of energy adequate to our needs at home and work and at the same time to control the costs of such energy and reduce the adverse effects of energy use, such as pollution and climate change. The supply-side approach to energy and environmental policy focuses on ensuring an adequate supply of energy by increasing its production and supply. Reform of such supply-side policy seeks to modify some aspects of energy supply to make them more economical or environmentally friendly—for example, by requiring emissions controls on automobiles, power plants, and residential, commercial, and industrial energy use, or by increasing the production and supply of energy from less costly or polluting sources, such as natural gas, nuclear power, or solar, wind, or hydro power. In contrast, demand-side energy and environmental policies seek to reduce the need, and hence the demand, for power through energy conservation, whether by making energy-using technologies (from light bulbs to cars) more energy-efficient or by reducing activities that consume nonrenewable energy, such as substituting mass transit or just plain walking for driving where possible.

The same synergy between supply and demand characterizes many other areas of policy. For example, reducing the use of problematic licit or illicit drugs can involve both attempts to control or block the supply of drugs and attempts to reduce demand by making people more aware of the harmful effects of drugs. National security can be sought by increasing the supply of military personnel and weapons while also reducing the need or demand for military force by addressing international tensions via diplomatic or economic trade policies.

Despite these familiar uses of both demand- and supply-side approaches in many major areas of public policy, health policy has been increasingly fixated on the supply side, and we seem to have become incapable of formulating a comprehensive demand-side alternative. Any policy area ultimately requires a judicious mix of supply-side and demand-side approaches. However, achieving such a balance in health policy will require a dramatically increased focus on demand-side policy.

Strategic Reason 2: The Need to Shift from Biomedical to Social Determinants of Health

The key to achieving a dramatic shift toward demand-side health policy, as we will see in chapter 3, is a fundamental strategic shift in how we think about the determinants of individual and population health—a shift in focus from biomedical determinants, though these cannot be forgotten, toward what are broadly termed social determinants, which include social, economic, environmental, behavioral, and psychological factors. *The social determinants provide the necessary lever for improving population health while reducing the need and demand, and hence expenditures, for health care and insurance.* This is a shift in thinking that has taken me my whole professional life to make. It will be similarly challenging for other individuals to grasp, and even more so for our larger society and public policy to comprehend and implement. Thus, we need to understand not only the scientific evidence that supports such a profound shift in thought and action but also the reasons we so naturally and doggedly persist in believing that health is simply, or certainly predominantly, a biomedical issue, and hence that health policy is essentially biomedical policy that should be largely concerned with health care and insurance.

To get to where we need to go—to achieve a shift toward demand-side health policy—we must understand not only where we are headed and why, but also the countervailing forces that will impede our movement in these directions.

Biological Limits on and Social Disparities in Health

It is also important to recognize that health is not like most other things that we seek to increase, many of which, notably most economic desiderata or goals, have no limits. There are no inherent limits on how much income or wealth an individual, organization, or society can achieve, which is not to say that their increase is easy or effortless, or even always desirable. Health, as we shall see in chapter 4, has real limits established by the evolutionary development of humans and other organisms over millennia. For example, though we all might wish to live forever—or at least the 969 years Methuselah is said to have lived—modern science suggests that human beings currently do not and cannot live beyond a maximum of about 125 years. This limit on life span—how long any person can maximally live—may not be immutable. However, increases in this limit have been, and will continue to be, much, much slower than improvements in how long people live on average (life expectancy) and how healthy they are while alive.

Life expectancy increased more in the nineteenth century than in all of prior history, and then did so again in the twentieth century—perhaps the most remarkable of all the achievements of human society. However, maximum biological life span increased, if at all, by only a small fraction of the gains in life expectancy and health. Similarly, there are also limits on how healthy and vital a human life can be, although again, such limits are not immutable. Given such limits, the goal of health practice and policy is to maximize the degree to which we are able to approach these limits as individuals and as a society—to live as long and as healthy as biologically possible.[7]

These biological limits on levels of individual and population health are critically important because some of us are much closer to approaching these limits than others. The socioeconomically advantaged among us are already approaching the biological limits—there is increasingly less that can be done to keep improving the length or health quality of their lives. There is much more opportunity, however, to improve the length and healthiness of life for those less economically fortunate, and they necessarily must be the focus of a demand-side approach to health policy. Hence, the problem of social disparities in health is central to health science and policy, not only as a matter of social justice, important as that is, but also in terms of developing a more rational, efficient, and effective health policy. Such a policy could not only improve health and reduce spending for health care and insurance but also add value to our economy and society through a more productive labor force and greater overall societal well-being.[8] Thus, chapter 4 will also focus on what we know about the changing nature of socioeconomic disparities in health and their implications for formulating a new demand-side health policy to resolve the paradoxical crisis of health care and health.

When people think and talk about social disparities in health, what first comes to mind are racial-ethnic and gender-based disparities more than socioeconomic ones. Chapter 5 will explore how and why socioeconomic disparities are fundamental to understanding racial-ethnic and gender disparities in health. It will also look at both the challenges and opportunities posed by race-ethnicity and gender—both separately and in combination with each other and with socioeconomic position—for a new demand-side approach to health and health policy.

Policy Implications

Once we recognize the fundamental importance of social determinants and disparities for health, and hence for health care utilization and expenditures, we can begin (in chapter 6) to envision what a demand-side approach to health education, research, and policy would look like and to find instances of it in current policies in the United States and abroad. We can also understand how redirecting money now focused on supply-side biomedical factors could pay for improving the social, economic, environmental, behavioral, and psychological conditions of life and work that promote health, including the public and private policies necessary to foster such conditions. Figure 1.1 suggests that 6 to 10 percent of GDP could be so redirected if our health expenditures were at the levels of other nations whose health is as good as or better than ours. All of these efforts can work hand-in-hand with efforts to reform the supply side of health policy and even facilitate such reform as people and policymakers recognize that very generous levels of health care and insurance are less important to their health than they have believed.[9] This recognition should make them less resistant to limiting care and insurance in various ways, and more appreciative of the health-promoting qualities of other "discretionary" nonhealth policy areas, such as education, income, macroeconomic, civil rights, housing/urban/neighborhood, agriculture, transportation, and environmental policy.

Two big issues need to be better understood and addressed if we are to realize the promise of a demand-side approach. First, we need to better understand *what, when, how,* and *for whom* nonhealth policies will be most effective in improving population health and reducing the need for health care utilization and expenditures. Chapter 7 explores what we know and can most appropriately apply toward these ends in the policy arena, both now and in future years. We need to evaluate more routinely the health effects of a wide range of nonhealth policies; where this has already been done, health impacts that rival or exceed those of major aspects of health care and insurance practice and policy have been found.

Second, we need to understand the ways and the extent to which improving population health and reducing social disparities in health can reduce health care utilization, and expenditures. Chapter 8 explores what we know about the actual and potential impacts of a healthier population on reducing expenditures for health care and insurance and on improving societal welfare and productivity. Existing research and projections indicate that a demand-side approach to health policy, which uses social determinants of health to reduce health disparities and improve population health, can improve population health and control and reduce spending for health care and insurance better than health care reform. Moreover, the potential expenditure reductions would be large enough to achieve current goals for reducing public and private expenditures for health care and insurance as part of the larger effort to bring overall levels of public and private debt under control.

Last, chapter 9 argues that the bankruptcy of our current policy and the limited potential impacts of any currently conceivable health care reforms compel us to seek new demand-side directions and policies for resolving America's paradoxical crisis of health and health care. Continuing to spend more and more on health care and insurance and getting less and less in terms of population health, not only relatively but perhaps even absolutely, is a disastrous recipe for both the actual and figurative health of our nation. Staying this course will not only fail to achieve the aims of better population health and lower expenditures on health but will eventually bankrupt our capacity to have meaningful and effective public policy in all other areas of our lives as well.

Conversely, better public policy in the discretionary nonhealth areas can improve population health, thereby reducing the need, demand, and expenditures for health care and insurance. We can hope that supply-side health care reform may also contribute to the simultaneous goals of improving population health and controlling expenditures for health care and insurance. But we cannot resolve our paradoxical crisis of spending more yet getting less without making a demand-side approach at least as central to health education, research, practice, and policy as current supply-side approaches. A demand-side approach to health policy promises not only to resolve America's paradoxical crisis of health and health care but also to provide the foundation for addressing the broader crisis of our society and public policy: our need to reverse a stifling buildup of public and private debt and infuse resources into the kind of public and private investment necessary to remain a major first-world country with good quality of life for all.

There is another way for American health policy to go if we can see our way clear to it. This book seeks to move us away from the knee-jerk supply-side policies that have cost us so much and given us so little in return and toward demand-side policies that, in addressing social determinants and disparities in health, will improve population health and reduce expenditures for health care and insurance. We have much to gain across the full range of public policy from beginning now to move steadily toward a demand-side approach to health policy.[10]

Part I

Historical and Scientific Foundations

Nothing that follows should be read as opposing health care and insurance or health care and insurance reform. We need the current reforms as much as we need a strong health care and insurance system, but they will not go far enough to resolve the paradoxical crisis of health care and health in this country. Moreover, our excessive focus and spending on health care and insurance run the risk of being counterproductive to the ends they seek to achieve.

Chapter 2

Health Care Reform: Necessary but Not Nearly Sufficient

The Patient Protection and Affordable Care Act of 2010 (hereafter ACA) is the most significant health care and insurance legislation since the establishment of Medicare and Medicaid almost fifty years ago. The overarching goal of this health care reform could be seen as resolving America's paradoxical crisis of health care and health, obviating the need for further major health policy legislation—and perhaps also the need for this book. However, the impact of this broad and dramatic legislation was significantly diminished by the negotiations and compromises necessary to its passage and is being further weakened in the continuing struggles over its implementation.[1]

Beyond these tactical problems, it is crucial to understand why it is strategically impossible to resolve America's paradoxical crisis through *any* process of health care and insurance reform, even a unitary single-payer system, much as such a system has to recommend it. Such "supply-side" policies and reforms, whether revolutionary or evolutionary, cannot alone, or even primarily, provide the kind of health policy needed to resolve America's paradoxical crisis of health care and health. At best, health care reform of the current ACA variety—or any currently conceivable variety—will have only marginal impacts on the two elements of America's paradox: rising health care expenditures and worsening population health. We will not understand the need for alternative demand-side solutions until we recognize this fact.

The Goals of Health Care Reform

Proponents of the ACA—and of almost all other proposals for health care reform debated during 2009 and 2010—had two major goals:

1. To provide universal access as much as possible to permanent and adequate health insurance for the American population
2. To reduce the level, or at least the rate of increase, of America's increasingly extraordinary level of expenditures for health care (see figure 1.1)

One or the other of these goals has often been more important to some proponents and constituencies, though recently controlling health care costs has become increasingly important for all. The almost complete focus of the Medicare/Medicaid legislation of 1965 on increasing access to health insurance resulted over the years in unanticipated levels of increased costs and expenditures. Thus, most subsequent health policy and legislation, including the ACA, has focused on reining in these costs.

Increasing access to care and insurance while simultaneously reducing expenditures on health care and insurance seem like contradictory goals. The ACA and other reform proposals with similar objectives have sought to overcome this seeming contradiction via a third goal: improving the quality and cost-effectiveness of health care and hence insurance. Accomplishing this third goal has involved trying to root out wasteful and ineffective health care utilization and spending, while promoting "evidence-based" care grounded in "comparative effectiveness" research that identifies the most cost-effective forms of preventive and therapeutic medical practice.

The success and impact of ACA, or any health care and insurance policy or reform, must be evaluated not only against these three goals—improving access to health care and insurance, controlling costs and expenditures, and improving the quality and cost-effectiveness of care—but also against a fourth overarching goal: *maintaining and improving individual and population health.* The success of the ACA and other supply-side approaches in achieving these goals is devoutly to be desired. However, the prognosis remains guarded; hence the need for new demand-side approaches and this book.

The Political and Economic Context of Health Care Reform

One only has to follow the political news out of Washington and the fifty states that bear major responsibility for implementing the Affordable Care Act to recognize how fragile are its prospects under current and foreseeable political and economic conditions. However, we also need to recognize an even more fundamental reality: we are unlikely, and arguably unable, to achieve any supply-side health care and insurance reform that will be deep and comprehensive enough to have a meaningful impact on either the seemingly inexorable rise of health care costs and expenditures or the alarming declines in population health relative to other nations, and perhaps even absolute for some portions of our population, that we have experienced over the last half-century. This unfortunate conclusion follows from the unchanging nature of both of these trends, graphically seen in figures 1.1 to 1.8, combined with all that we understand theoretically and empirically about the political and economic context of the American health care and insurance system.

American Exceptionalism in Health Policy

America is the only highly developed country in the world without a nationally integrated system of health care and insurance. The United States is also exceptional among wealthy developed countries in the degree to which its social welfare system is relatively equally divided between the public and private sectors. This is most evident in retirement pensions and health care and insurance, two areas that account for the largest part of social welfare spending in all wealthy developed countries and hence also constitute the crux of current efforts to address the debt crisis afflicting both the public and private sectors in North American and European nations.[2]

The United States is often viewed as an impoverished welfare state, but this is true only if we consider social welfare spending in the public sector. By a series of policy decisions over many decades, the United States has assigned to the private sector much of the responsibility for what are largely public governmental responsibilities in all other wealthy developed nations, most notably health care and insurance and old-age pensions. If we add this private-sector spending to that of the public sector, the United States looks about average in total social welfare spending among comparable nations.

However, this divided structure of the welfare state, which has been advanced and reinforced for at least a century, makes our health care and insurance system increasingly intractable to reform. It has created a growing panoply of large and powerful private groups with vested interests in the status quo. These interest groups range from doctors and hospitals to insurance companies and provider organizations, to pharmaceutical and medical equipment suppliers and manufacturers, and even in some times and places to labor unions. Which of these interest groups is most powerful and active in maintaining the status quo has changed over time: from doctors and hospitals in the 1930s through the 1960s, to pharmaceutical and other manufacturers in the 1990s, to insurance companies today. These interest groups have repeatedly blocked efforts to significantly modify the American employer-based health care and insurance system, except for the poor and the old, who are relatively unprofitable to insure; and these groups have strongly shaped even Medicare and Medicaid programs to benefit private as well as public interests.[3]

The Likely Effects of the Affordable Care Act

Given these conditions, the passage of the Affordable Care Act was in many ways a remarkable political accomplishment, though achieved at substantial cost to the Obama administration and Democratic congressional majorities. The ACA has increased Americans' access to health care and insurance and will continue to do so. However, both the immediate tactical problems of implementation and the long-term and strategic problems discussed in this chapter make it likely that ACA, at best, will only marginally move the status quo of health and health care in America toward the goals of better health, lower costs and expenditures, and more efficient and cost-effective health care.

Access to Care

Prior to state opposition to insurance exchanges and Medicaid expansion, ACA had been expected to cover about two-thirds of those without health insurance in any given year (or about 30 million of the approximately 50 million currently not covered). It will still undoubtedly advance considerably toward this goal. And insurance will be more adequate and stable for all. Beyond improving access to health care for many, this is a major achievement for two other reasons. First, it provides a firmer foundation for efforts to control costs, which become easier the more universal the coverage of any insurance system. Second, it will facilitate making health care more evidence-based and cost-effective on a broader scale since insurance reimbursement systems constitute a major lever for creating change in health care practice.

Levels of Individual and Population Health

Most proponents of health care reform, especially those seeking more universal insurance coverage and access to health insurance and care, expect such reform and access to significantly improve the health of both those acquiring new access to insurance and care and the American population as a whole. For several reasons, however, they are likely to be disappointed by ACA or any other reform creating more universal access to health insurance and care. First, those Americans without health insurance are not just, or even mainly, those who are most socioeconomically disadvantaged or most in need of care; Medicare, Medicaid, and Children's Health Insurance Plans already cover many such individuals.

Many of the uninsured who gain coverage under ACA will be members of relatively healthy parts of the population, including young adults and many workers (and their dependents) whose employers do not provide health insurance benefits. Mandatory coverage for such persons does more to increase the affordability of insurance for all than it does to improve the health of the previously uninsured. Finally, many uninsured do receive care when seriously in need, albeit often less efficient and less effective care. What ACA does is make health care more readily and steadily available for all, with clear benefits for people with "preexisting conditions" such as hypertension and diabetes that require regular sustained care to prevent or postpone the development of more serious morbidity or mortality. These are important and valuable benefits, but the number of such people is not large enough to have substantial effects on overall population health.

These guarded expectations are largely confirmed by the best available empirical evidence to date. A variety of studies that control well for sociodemographic differences between the insured and uninsured (in terms of age, sex, race-ethnicity, and socioeconomic level) find generally small or even zero impacts of health insurance on health despite increased utilization of care.[4] Similarly, major changes in national health policy (such as the introduction of national health care or insurance programs in the United Kingdom in 1948, in Canada in 1970, and in the United States in 1965) have not produced major shifts in levels of or trends in population health that are clearly attributable to the effects of health care or insurance.

And the evidence from the only major randomized experiments in providing health insurance to the uninsured in the United States has shown similarly small and limited impacts on health. The RAND Health Insurance Experiment, completed in 1982, focused on evaluating the impact of varying levels of copayment on health care utilization and expenditures. It showed that cost-sharing reduces health services utilization, and hence expenditures, without "significantly affecting the quality of care" or "participant health." Those receiving free care, however, showed modest and selective improvements in health "among the poorest and sickest 6 percent of the sample at the start of the experiment."[5] A recent randomized study of another relatively unhealthy population—new Social Security Disability Insurance beneficiaries—similarly found increased health care utilization, "fewer unmet needs," lower out-of-pocket health care spending, and "reported-improved health" among those who received Medicare insurance immediately versus having to wait twenty-nine months to become Medicare-eligible, as required by current law.[6] Finally, a randomized study of Medicaid expansion in Oregon—quite analogous to what will occur under ACA in states that choose to participate—found "that Medicaid coverage generated no significant improvements in measured physical health outcomes in the first two years, but it did increase use of health care services, raise rates of diabetes detection and management, lower rates of depression, and reduce financial strain."[7] Note that, across these studies, insurance may have greater economic benefits (reduced out-of-pocket spending and financial strain) than health benefits.

Several non-experimental studies have recently estimated the health impact of the Massachusetts health care reform of 2006, the state-level precursor and analogue of the ACA.[8] These studies have several advantages: larger samples, the inclusion of a number of health indicators, and a longer follow-up period, generally more than four to four and a half years. They have two disadvantages, however: they are non-experimental (comparing changes in Massachusetts to those in comparison counties or states in the United States or New England), and they rely largely on self-reported data from the Behavioral Risk Factors Surveillance System telephone survey and, in one case, county-level mortality data. Nevertheless, the results are largely consistent with the experimental studies: the non-experimental studies find generally small improvements in health among Massachusetts residents post-reform compared with other states or U.S. counties, and improvements that are larger among less healthy and/or socially disadvantaged portions of that population. They also find somewhat larger increases in both health care utilization and spending post-reform in Massachusetts relative to other states or counties.

Figure 2.1 shows the potential effects of the 2006 Massachusetts health care reforms on mortality from a quasi-experimental comparison over time between Massachusetts and a matched pool of counties from across the United States. As in other studies, the observed differences are modest to small, and not definitively a function of health insurance alone. In the words of the authors: "In absolute terms we found a decrease in mortality [in Massachusetts relative to the control group] of .00082 percentage points with an increase in coverage of 6.8 percentage points, which implies that for approximately every 830 adults who gained insurance, there was 1 fewer death per year. . . . It is possible that the post reform reduction in mortality in Massachusetts was due to other factors such as the [Great Recession]. . . . The extent to which our results generalize to the United States . . . is unclear."[9]

Health Care Costs and Expenditures

The ACA arguably contains virtually all promising ideas for restraining the growth of total health care utilization and expenditures and increasing their cost-effectiveness. However, because of the strength and influence of a medical-biotechnology complex with vested interests in maintaining or increasing health care utilization and expenditures—from

Figure 2.1 Unadjusted Mortality Rates for Adults Age Twenty to Sixty-Four in Massachusetts Versus a Control Group, 2001–2010

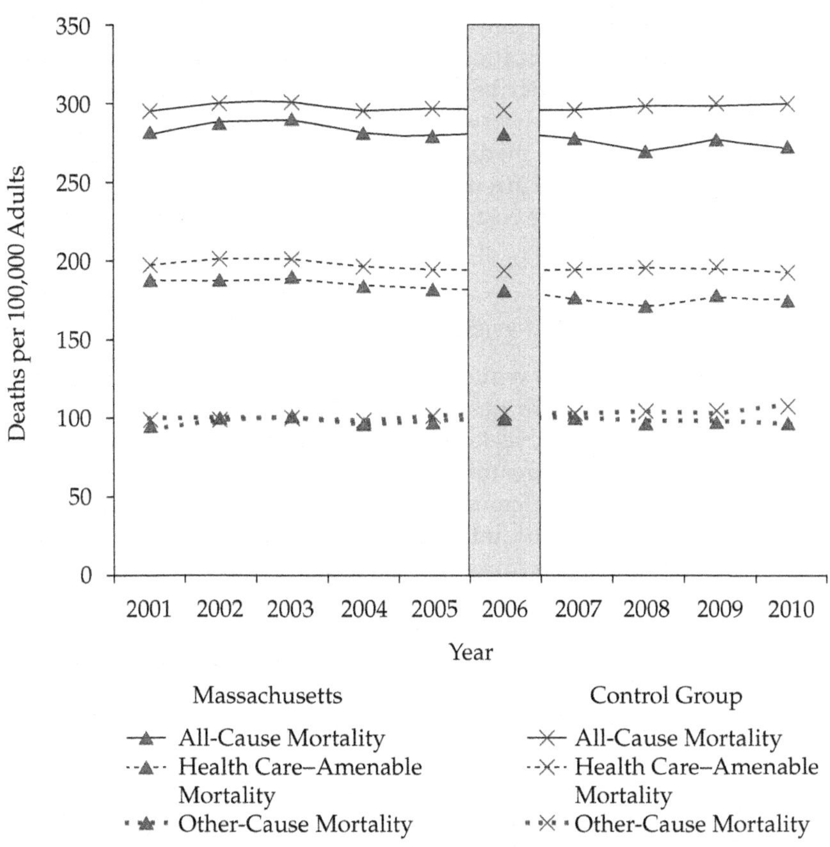

Source: Sommers et al. (2014). © 2014 The American College of Physicians. Reprinted with permission.

Note: The shaded band designates the beginning of the Massachusetts state health care reform which was implemented starting in July 2006. "Health care–amenable mortality" is as defined in table 1 of the supplement [to the article]. "Other-cause mortality" covers all other causes of death not included in that definition.

health care providers to hospitals, to producers of medical devices, technology, and drugs, to private health insurers (and perhaps even public ones in and of themselves)—we simply cannot expect currently envisaged reform efforts to greatly reduce unnecessary access to or provision of health care or to substantially limit the costs and expenditures associated with health care. The largely inexorable growth of health care spending in the United States over the last forty to fifty years, despite repeated efforts to control it through both broader and more focused health care and insurance reform and regulation, confirms this expectation. Momentarily successful efforts—such as the development of fixed or "bundled" payments for hospital care of specific types of problems (diagnostically related groups and "prospective payment" in Medicare), or the use of health maintenance organizations and increased gatekeeping by primary care providers—have either been eroded over time by push-back from patients and providers or overwhelmed by other forces, such as increasingly complex and costly medical technology, resulting in more expensive forms of care. Thus, current forecasts and projections about the impact of ACA on health care costs and expenditures tend to average out to around zero.[10]

Improving the Cost-Effectiveness of Care

The main hope for ACA to reduce health care costs and expenditures and improve population health lies in its smaller and more detailed provisions. These, for example, seek to promote research on the comparative effectiveness of medical treatments, deepen the focus on primary care and prevention, and implement more uniform and "evidence-based" standards of care, aided by information technology. To the extent that they are successful, such efforts could markedly improve the quality of care on a large scale and reduce its costs at the margins. In spite of their great promise, however, it remains uncertain whether we can implement these innovations on a broad enough scale to realize their potential benefits for improving health and reducing health care spending. Electronic health records (EHRs), for example, are one of the centerpieces of ACA's efforts to improve quality of care, but their ability to do so is currently in question.[11] And again, on balance, even if all of these innovations realize the fondest hopes of their proponents, their health impact will be modest—albeit beneficial—because, as we will see in chapter 3, health care is not the major determinant of health.[12] Moreover, the substantial inertia as well as active opposition to reform in America's large, exceptional, and quite decentralized system of health care and insurance is very likely to continue and will only further moderate the potential gains in improving the cost-effectiveness of care.[13]

Conclusion

Any sector of the economy that is approaching 20 percent of total gross domestic product needs to be made as cost-effective as possible, especially a sector, like health, that partially constitutes and heavily affects human well-being. Thus, efforts at health care and insurance reform will continue to be necessary as one means to that goal. However, we need to be hard-headedly realistic—rather than idealistically, or even illusorily,

Box 2.1 Probable Effects of the ACA

1.	Access to health insurance and care	Substantially positive
2.	Quality and cost-effectiveness of care	Potentially very positive, but probably modestly so
3.	Levels of population health	Marginally positive
4.	Health care costs and expenditures	Uncertain and at best marginally positive

optimistic—regarding the extent to which such supply-side health policy reform is capable of achieving its goals. Based on all available understanding and evidence of the nature and functioning of the health care and insurance system in the past, present, and future, box 2.1 summarizes the probable effects of the ACA—or any currently conceivable supply-side reform of the American health care and insurance system—with respect to the goals that have been articulated for such reform.

The probable outcomes are ordered here from greatest and most positive to smallest and least positive. ACA and most other proposals for health care reform seek, and will achieve, the expansion of access to health insurance and health care for more Americans. Many regard this as furthering a fundamental human right, and almost all would regard this as desirable for improving health and controlling the costs and expenditures associated with health care and insurance. However, for the reasons discussed in this chapter as well as in chapter 3, increased access to health insurance and care is likely to affect both population health and health spending only at the margins. Much the same can be said about the goals of increasing the quality and cost-effectiveness of medical care: these are necessary and desirable goals that are likely to be achieved to some degree, but probably only moderately, and with generally marginal effects on overall levels of population health and health care costs and expenditures.

The reasons for these modest impacts of reform lie not only in the nature of America's exceptional, and in many ways dysfunctional, system of health care and insurance but equally or more in the fundamental misunderstanding that underlies American health policy: the assumption that health care is the major determinant of population health. Chapter 3 addresses the population health impacts of medical care, which, though real and much to be desired, are actually rather limited. While examining why we persist in believing otherwise, the chapter also delineates what are in fact the major determinants of population health. These insights, along with those regarding social disparities in health in chapters 4 and 5, open the way for thinking about a new demand-side approach to health policy. Such an approach offers greater promise for resolving America's paradoxical crisis of health care and health—and hence for realizing the major goals of health care reform—than does health care reform itself, desirable and important as such reform remains as one component of a broader and deeper change in health policy for America.

Chapter 3

Health Care ≠ Health: From Biomedical to Social Determinants of Health

WE HAVE remained fixated for a century or more on the notion that health policy is essentially health care and insurance policy, and hence that reform or improvement of health policy can only be addressed via health care and insurance reform. This fixation derives from an underlying belief that health care is the predominant determinant of health and therefore the way to maintain and improve individual and population health is to provide more universal access to more and better health care. Thus, all major health policy legislation, from Medicare and Medicaid in the mid-1960s to the Affordable Care Act (ACA) of 2010, has been focused on these goals—leavened increasingly by the seemingly contradictory goal of reducing the utilization of and expenditures for medical care.[1]

We cannot get beyond these beliefs without understanding why we hold to them so completely and tenaciously, even as scientific evidence mounts that they are incomplete and often mistaken. Only then can we begin to put these beliefs in proper perspective and move on to develop a complementary demand-side approach to health policy—which offers much better prospects of achieving the major goals of supply-side health care reform and resolving our paradoxical crisis of spending more and more on health care and insurance and getting less and less in terms of population health.

Why We Think Health (Policy) = Health Care and Insurance (Policy)

The "we" in the heading of this section is meant quite intentionally to include myself. Here and in later chapters, I reflect on my own life and health to illustrate some of the issues I discuss. I hope that this approach not only proves useful in its own right but also helps and encourages readers to think about the broad issues of health science and policy addressed in this book in relation to their own lives and experience.

To begin, I confess that it has taken me all my life to get beyond the conventional wisdom that health is primarily a function of health care, and hence that health policy is primarily health care and insurance policy. So I do not expect it to be easy for others—both individually and, even more, collectively—to question this assumption. But get beyond it we must, and the sooner the better. I hope that the insights that have influenced and changed me can help others to do the same. So let us begin with why we all find it so natural to believe that health care is what drives and determines health.

Health Care Important for Health, but Less Than We Think

Even the most seriously flawed beliefs often reflect some grain of truth. It is certainly true that health care plays an important part in shaping individual and population health. We all know this from personal experience and are thankful to have access to good health care when we need it. As an adult, my life has been improved, extended, and perhaps already saved by the ability to control my blood pressure via a single, modest-dosage daily tablet of antihypertensive medication, with virtually no side effects.

Similarly, much scientific evidence documents the benefits of preventive and therapeutic health care for health. And if we place a monetary value on human life and health, economic analyses suggest, there is a positive return, at least on average, from even our current high expenditures for health care and insurance.[2]

This is not to say, however, that health care is the *most* important determinant of health in individuals and especially in populations, or that the health returns on investments in health care and insurance are very cost-effective, either absolutely or relative to other potential means of creating, maintaining, and enhancing health. Quite the contrary. Since 1980, as relative and even absolute levels of population health have worsened, the health spending required to achieve a gain of one year of life expectancy has increased, especially at older ages.[3] The fact is that many other factors on which we often spend much less than on health care and insurance, both individually and collectively, have as great or greater positive effects, dollar for dollar, on our health. These nonmedical factors will be examined in this and later chapters.

Yet a near-religious faith in the benefits of health care has led us to devote almost 20 percent of our gross domestic product (GDP) to it and to recoil from almost any suggestion that we reduce our access to and utilization of care, whether via "death panels" or limitations on access to medical specialists. Neither our personal experiences with the health care system nor the scientific evidence of its positive effects on health can alone account for such a strong and persistent faith and associated body of conventional wisdom. Much more is involved—psychologically, culturally, socially, and institutionally.

Psychological Attribution Errors and Biases

Psychology has shown that we are all naive scientists trying to develop causal theories or attributions for what we observe in the world so that we can behave more effectively. But as *naive* scientists, we have not mastered the self-correcting procedures that actual scientists use (for example, experimental design or statistical estimation and adjustment) to protect against the kinds of errors in information processing that make ordinary mortals susceptible to bias in causal attributions. One of the most powerfully biasing tendencies of the average person is to give undue weight to a particularly prominent or dramatic cause or event relative to a larger body of less prominent or dramatic evidence.[4]

In my own life, two examples stand out: the elimination of polio in this country and many others (but sadly, not yet in all), and the power of selected surgical and pharmacological treatments. Poliomyelitis, a fatal or severely paralytic or functionally limiting disease, struck in epidemic proportions of 50,000 or more cases in the United States in 1952. Until I was ten years old, my brother and I and our parents, like most other children and parents and young adults at that time, avoided swimming pools and other crowded public places every summer, in fear of contracting this dreaded disease. Between the summers of 1954 and 1955, however, that fear was virtually eradicated, along with poliomyelitis itself, by the discovery and epidemiologic demonstration of a safe and effective vaccine against polio.

Even more dramatic than the impact of the polio vaccine are the "healing miracles" of modern medicine that we have all experienced. I am not only grateful for the excellent control of my blood pressure produced by a single little daily pill, but still recall with wonder taking the first pill and having my systolic blood pressure drop, within a half-hour, by about twenty points and my diastolic by about ten—dropping, that is, to essentially normal levels.[5] Similarly, an appendectomy at age twenty put an instant end to the acute appendicitis that had painfully interrupted my holiday weekend in New York City. And I still remember the family doctor coming to my house when I was about five and prescribing Aureomycin, the first of the tetracycline antibiotics. Within twenty-four hours, the medication (which cost, as I recall, a then-astronomical $1 per pill) almost miraculously transformed me from a very sick little boy into a healthy one.

The ability of biomedical science to produce dramatic cures in individuals and in broader populations leads to a tendency to see that science, and the health care deriving from it, as more potent and effective than it really is on average. We often forget or fail to recognize the equal or greater number of instances in which the care prescribed or given was not the reason we were cured or healed (most viruses run their course without treatment, and sometimes it is the placebo effect of being treated that helps), was simply ineffective (my only case of pneumonia was not correctly diagnosed and treated until the third try, by then at much greater cost and with a much slower recovery time), or was even sometimes iatrogenic (as with the side effects of drugs like thalidomide and Vioxx).

Further, when an antibiotic or vaccine cures us or inoculates us against one infectious disease, we tend to believe that the same or similar antibiotics and vaccines can do likewise against other diseases. Thus, we even tend to pressure health care professionals to give us drugs (and even surgeries) that they forewarn us are not likely to work, and we support the search for pharmaceutical, surgical, and even genetic treatments for any and all health problems—including behaviors, such as smoking and immoderate consumption of alcohol or food, that we come to define as "medical" problems rather than as the social and psychological problems that they really are.

The call for *evidence-based medicine* as part of health care reform is an attempt to correct our attributional biases, but health care professionals (many of whom value their "clinical experience and judgment" over statistical evidence) as well as patients often find this antidote hard to accept. In addition to all of our "normal" attributional biases, we are bombarded by journalistic accounts of medical breakthroughs, but the media pay much less attention to the many treatments that are tried but not effective and tend to inform us about only the most serious of iatrogenic practices.

Broader Cultural Beliefs, Spurious Correlations, and the Biomedical Paradigm

Even when we try to attend to a broad array of data or evidence, we still may develop strongly held and biased beliefs through a mechanism that scientists and statisticians label "spurious or illusory correlation"—making erroneous causal inferences from a correlation we observe. A classic example appears in statistics textbooks: observing the number of fire trucks at a fire and the damage caused by the fire, we are likely to find a strong positive correlation between them. Obviously, however, this correlation does not mean that fire trucks cause fire damage, or that setting a fire will produce a fire truck; rather, the number of fire trucks and the amount of damage are both caused by a third factor—the size of the fire.

Our strong belief in the power of biomedical professionals, knowledge, and spending to produce health is driven by an analogous and broader, if more complex, form of spurious correlation. Probably the largest and most important change in the history of human life and society has been the increase in human life expectancy—from about thirty years in the late eighteenth century to almost seventy years on average for the world today, and eighty or more years in the most developed nations. Between the late eighteenth century and the beginning of the twentieth century, human life expectancy increased by more than it had in all prior human history, which had added only five to ten years to the average twenty-five-year life expectancy of prehistoric humans. Between the late nineteenth century and the beginning of the twenty-first, life expectancy increased again more than in all of prior human history. Barring some major genetic transformation of the human race, human health and longevity are unlikely to improve so rapidly again as life expectancy approaches the biological limit of the average human life span that has evolved since the origins of humankind—around 110 years (see chapter 4).

For most of us, the single major development most correlated with this rise in human life expectancy is the rise of modern biomedical science and health care over the same time period. The introduction of a relatively safe and effective polio vaccine in 1954 capped a series of triumphs from the late eighteenth century through the mid-twentieth century in the use of vaccines, antibiotics, and prophylactic agents, from antiseptics to pesticides, to prevent, treat, and even virtually eradicate many forms of infectious disease. The result was a widely shared belief in a biomedical model of health grounded in the doctrine of "specific etiology"—the theory that each disease has a specific biological cause that can be identified and then effectively treated, prevented, or eradicated by modern biomedical science and practice. Although this theory is valid in some ways for many diseases and in most ways for a few, we will see that it is based on spurious or illusory correlation with respect to much or most of the improvement in human health during this time period—and even more so with respect to the changes in human health that emerged during a new era of chronic disease in the last half of the twentieth century in developed countries, and increasingly in developing societies as well.

Social and Institutional Reinforcers of Individual Psychology and Collective Belief

The psychological and cultural processes and beliefs underlying the assumption that health is a product of biomedical research and practice came to be embodied over the last half of the twentieth century in a set of increasingly large and powerful social institutions: the health service professions, hospitals, biomedical research institutions, pharmaceutical organizations, and insurance companies. These institutions believed in the biomedical paradigm of health, and they also benefited enormously—in terms of money, power, and prestige—from supporting and disseminating that paradigm among the broader population. This institutional reinforcement of the biomedical paradigm created further barriers to health care reform and alternative paradigms for thinking about health.

These barriers went beyond individual psychology and collective cultural beliefs to include socioeconomic structures and processes and political power. The medical-biotechnology complex is now larger than the military-industrial complex ever was, and it is powerful enough to have made the United States, for example, the only nation in which prescription drugs and medical procedures can be advertised via TV, radio, the Internet, newspapers, and magazines. These sociopolitical and economic forces reinforce psychological and cultural factors, overdetermining the systems of thought and action that have equated health (policy) with health care and insurance (policy).

The Emergence of the Dominant Biomedical Paradigm in the Late Nineteenth and Early Twentieth Centuries

These mutually reinforcing forces predispose, and almost constrain, us to believe that biomedical science and the health care deriving from it are the most powerful determinants of human health. It is thus little wonder that by the mid-twentieth century this biomedical paradigm had become dominant in health science and policy and deeply ingrained in popular consciousness and culture. Hence, our individual and collective approaches to health have remained fixed on expanding the quantity and quality of biomedical science and access to it via clinical practice. This approach to health science, practice, and policy represents, however, only one understanding of the forces shaping individual and population health, albeit one that became dominant and has had considerable utility in its time and place. To better understand, evaluate, and reinterpret this approach in our current time and situation, we must go back to the mid-nineteenth century, when this approach was born.[6]

Health Care and Health in the Nineteenth Century

In the mid-nineteenth century, there was no dominant approach to understanding human health and disease and hence to promoting the former and combating the latter. Nor was there any systematic base of scientific evidence for choosing between competing forms of medical science and practice—osteopathy versus homeopathy versus the ultimately triumphant allopathic medicine. In the area of public health, there was a growing body of practice, dating back to ancient times and revived by social reformers such as Edwin Chadwick, aimed at promoting hygiene and cleanliness in housing, clothing, public places, air quality, water supply and use, and the disposal of waste and sewage. But these practices were grounded in unsubstantiated theories of "miasmas" or general filth as the major threats to health, though these theories contained some grains of truth.[7]

Even in scientific academic medicine, Rudolf Virchow, the German physician and liberal politician generally viewed as the founder of modern cellular pathology, developed the early foundations of what has come to be termed "social medicine." In studying the spread of infectious disease, most notably typhus in Silesia in the 1840s, Virchow argued that socioeconomic factors, especially poverty, drive the spread of infectious disease. In the revolutionary year of 1848, Virchow wrote, "Medicine is a social science and politics is nothing but medicine on a grand scale."[8]

The Rise of Bacteriology and Modern Biomedical Science

Both the multiplicity of perspectives on health and medicine and the incipient social medicine of the mid-nineteenth century were radically altered and rapidly transcended by the development of modern bacteriology and virology over the course of the nineteenth century. The work of Edward Jenner, Louis Pasteur, Robert Koch, and others grounded the science, medical prevention, and treatment of infectious diseases in a basic biological science of pathogenic infectious organisms spread via human and animal contact and vectors such as air, water, and food. This new science seemed to render prior knowledge and understandings of health and disease largely obsolete. As early as 1890, the first Nobel Laureate in Medicine, Emil Behring, dismissed the research and writing on social medicine of Rudolf Virchow and others: "While these views . . . had their merits [in 1848], now, following the procedure of Robert Koch, the study of infectious disease can be pursued unswervingly without being sidetracked by social considerations and reflections on social policy."[9]

Over the decades of the late nineteenth and early twentieth centuries, the hegemony of this biomedical paradigm, which sees each disease as having a specific cause that can be identified and countered by vaccination/inoculation or treatment, came to dominate medical science, education, and practice, including much of public health as well. The steady decline of infectious disease and the coincident increase in life expectancy seemed to provide empirical support for the validity and utility of the biomedical paradigm in medicine and public health.

The Flexner Report and Modern Medical Education

The biomedical paradigm became the foundation of medical education in the United States in the first decade of the twentieth century. In 1904 the American Medical Association, the professional association of allopathic medical practitioners, created the Council of Medical Education (CME). CME defined proper medical education as two years of training in anatomy and physiology followed by two years of clinical training in a teaching hospital. In 1908 it commissioned a study of American medical schools by the Carnegie Foundation for the Advancement of Teaching, which chose an educator, Abraham Flexner, to carry out the study. The Flexner Report of 1910 endorsed the CME's recommended curriculum and recommended that admission to American medical schools require a high school diploma and at least two years of college or university study, primarily devoted to basic science. It also recommended closing many existing medical schools and incorporating the remaining ones into larger universities.[10]

Though the Flexner Report may have merely codified ongoing trends and development, that codification remains the foundation of medical education, and hence research and practice. It greatly professionalized and improved the practice of medicine in many ways, but as Behring had advocated two decades earlier, it also institutionalized the separation of health education, research, practice, and policy from broader social and political education, research, practice, and policy. In so doing, it cast aside not only a great deal of quackery and unscientific theory and practice in medicine but also the tradition carried on by Virchow, Chadwick, and others of pursuing systematic work on the broader social determinants of health to find sociopolitical ways to promote health and prevent disease.[11]

Onward to the Mid-Twentieth Century

The rise and success of modern biomedical research, education, and practice continued largely unabated through the first half of the twentieth century. Infectious disease declined even further, and astonishing improvements in health and life expectancy remained the order of the day, at least in the developed nations of the world, even in the face of two world wars and the Great Depression. The biomedical paradigm arguably reached its high-water mark with the quite stunning virtual eradication of polio in developed countries in the years immediately following the successful field trials of the Salk vaccine in 1954; this success followed upon the increasingly widespread and effective use of antibiotics to treat many infectious diseases. By the 1960s, however, other developments were under way that would eventually challenge, but also complement, the dominant biomedical paradigm.

A Growing Recognition of Non-Biomedical Determinants of Health

During my formal education, I never had a course that even entertained, much less seriously explored, a role for non-biomedical factors in understanding the nature and etiology of physical health or finding ways to promote health and control disease. Indeed, no such courses were offered in either the undergraduate or graduate institutions that I attended in the 1960s, excellent as they were. Only at the end of that decade, in my dissertation work, did I learn that there was a developing science of health based equally or more in social and behavioral sciences and their intersections with biology and physiology. Four decades later, I see four major lines of development that began at that time and that continue to provide the foundation for new approaches to health research, practice, and policy.

The Epidemiologic Transition

The first of these developments was a change in the nature of disease in human populations—widely known as the "epidemiologic transition"—which first came to prominence in the United States and other developed countries in the 1950s and 1960s.[12] As human life expectancy grew with the decline of infectious disease, people became more susceptible to diseases whose etiology and course developed over decades rather than days and hence only became prevalent as people's average life expectancy began to extend into their fifties and sixties over the first half of the twentieth century. By the 1950s and 1960s, chronic diseases, especially cardiovascular disease and cancer, became "epidemic" in the United States and other developed countries, and gradually in many developing ones as well. From the late 1950s to the late 1960s, the growing dominance of chronic disease slowed, and then virtually halted, especially among men, the two-century-long increase in life expectancy that had characterized the nations of North America and Western Europe since the mid-eighteenth century. Modern biomedical science, as it had developed to that point, seemed momentarily immobilized and powerless to arrest, much less roll back, these new epidemics.

Risk Factors: Biological, Environmental, Behavioral, and Psychosocial

Chronic diseases are chronic in both their etiology and their course. Diseases like heart disease and cancer stem from processes that develop and operate over decades before becoming manifest or symptomatic. And people are not generally, if ever, "cured" of such diseases. Rather, they live with these diseases for years and even decades before they become disabling or fatal. Such a long-term development and course of illness, almost by definition, cannot be a function of a single etiologic agent—such as a bacterium, virus, or even gene—that can be countered by a single prophylactic or therapeutic "magic bullet." Instead, these diseases reflect the cumulative, and frequently synergistic, interaction of multiple factors operating over substantial periods of time, with no single factor either necessary or sufficient to produce disease. The "causal," or at least predictive, power of these factors is probabilistic: singly or in combination, they increase the *risk* for developing a chronic disease. Thus, a new terminology—"risk factors"—emerged to denote these multiple, contingent, causal factors in chronic disease. And a new methodology was developed to identify them: the long-term prospective observational study.[13] The prototype of such a study is the Framingham Heart Study, which has sought to medically examine and track, over decades, the adult population of Framingham, Massachusetts, to identify factors that predict the onset of cardiovascular disease.[14]

At first, the search for risk factors remained focused on biomedical variables such as blood pressure and blood lipids, especially cholesterol, as well as subclinical indicators of heart or lung damage or dysfunction that could be identified by new procedures and tests, such as X-rays and electrocardiograms. These risk factors have remained the core biomedical variables for preventing, detecting, and treating cardiovascular disease to this day. However, the web of risk factors gradually began to widen to include environmental, behavioral, and eventually psychosocial risk factors. Beginning in the 1950s and 1960s, many chemicals, along with physical substances such as soot, asbestos, coal dust, and general airborne particulate matter and pollution, and even something as seemingly benign as sunlight, were increasingly recognized as major risk factors and causal agents for cancer, as well as for respiratory and cardiovascular diseases. At the same time, behavioral factors such as diet, alcohol use, and levels of physical activity and exercise began to draw attention as potential risk (or protective) factors, especially for cardiovascular disease. Particularly notable for the breadth and depth of its health effects was the behavior of cigarette smoking.

First in Great Britain and then in the United States via the 1964 Surgeon General's report on smoking and health, cigarette smoking was shown to be a major cause of lung and other respiratory cancers, as well as cardiovascular and other diseases.[15] Indeed, as shown in figure 3.1, both cigarette smoking and respiratory cancer were almost nonexistent in the early twentieth century. Cigarette smoking grew dramatically over the first half of the century, peaking in the 1950s and 1960s, then gradually but steadily declined to the present level in response to increasing efforts to curb smoking in the wake of the Surgeon General's report. With the lag of twenty to thirty years that it takes smoking to have its carcino-

Figure 3.1 Cigarette Consumption and Respiratory Cancer Mortality, 1900–2006

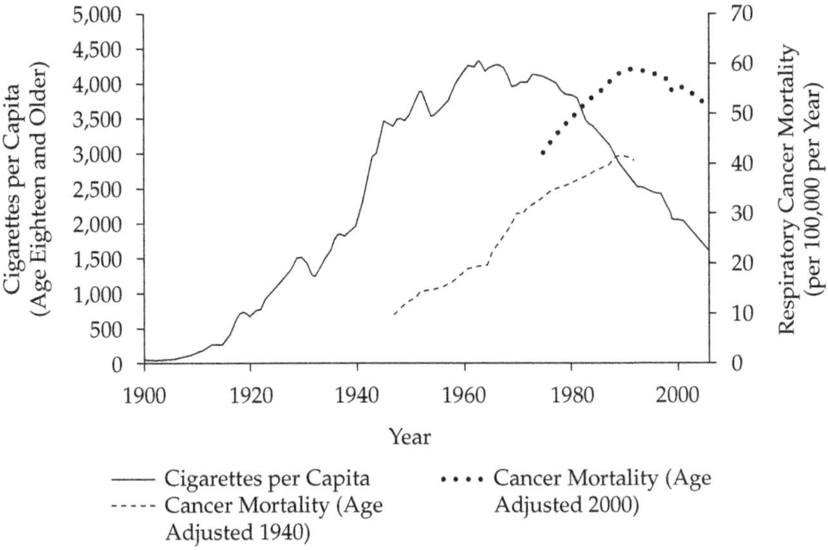

Sources: Author compilation based on Young (1998, 200); Centers for Disease Control and Prevention, Smoking and Tobacco Use Consumption Data (2015); and National Cancer Institute Surveillance, Epidemiology, and End Results (SEER) (1975–2007).

genic effects, respiratory cancer rates rose from the 1930s to the 1990s and have now begun a gradual but steady decline.

The clear evidence that smoking is a major risk factor for mortality spurred the development of still-growing fields of research into other health behaviors, or "lifestyles," especially the roles of physical activity and moderate eating (and weight), and alcohol consumption in promoting health and preventing disease. The risk factor status of these behaviors gradually became accepted in biomedical and other scientific circles, leading to major public health and policy initiatives against smoking and eventually a range of other deleterious health behaviors, including obesity.

The range of risk factors grew to include more psychosocial risk factors, from chronic and acute stress to psychological dispositions to social relationships and supports. Perhaps most striking and consistent was the evidence from multiple Framingham-like prospective studies, as shown in figure 3.2, that social isolation, or a low level of social integration (relationships or ties), is associated, especially among men, with the same doubling of risk for mortality from all causes as cigarette smoking. Simi-

Figure 3.2 Social Integration and Age-Adjusted Mortality for Males in Prospective Studies, 1960s to 1980s

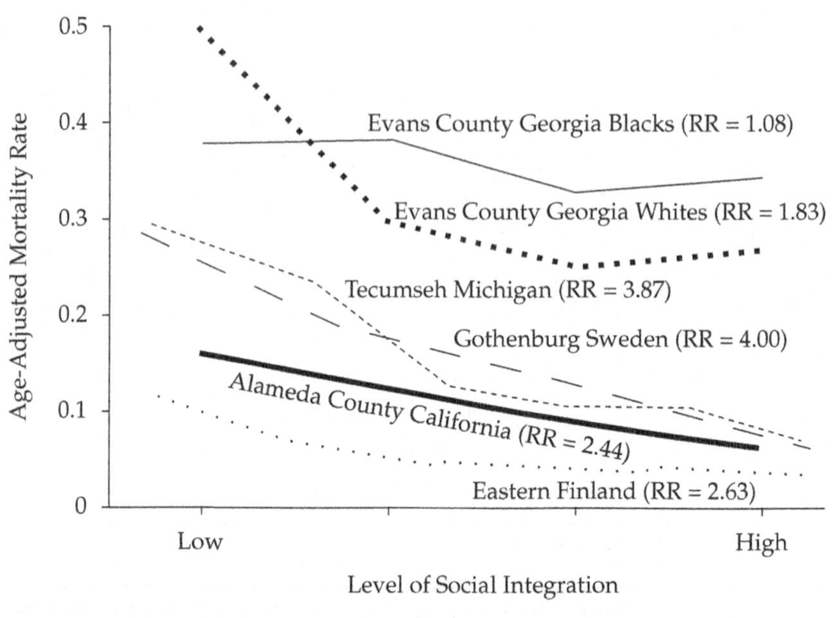

Source: House et al. (1988, figure 1).
Note: RR equals the relative risk ratio of mortality at the lowest versus highest level of social integration.

lar results were obtained for psychosocial stress and a number of psychological traits, dispositions, or "behavior patterns."[16]

How Psychosocial Factors "Get Under the Skin"

Beginning in the early part of the twentieth century and accelerating after World War II, theory and laboratory evidence were developed to explain how and why phenomena that seem purely social and psychological can induce major changes in key physiologic systems (nervous, endocrine, cardiovascular, and gastrointestinal), such as a rise in blood pressure or cholesterol. If prolonged, these changes can produce actual chronic disease—such as hypertension and its sequelae in cardiovascular and renal disease—and even death. Such psychophysiological theories of "stress" were later joined by the new field of psychoneuroimmunology, which showed and explained how psychosocial stressors and deprivations can depress or disrupt the operation of the immune system, increasing the risk of infectious and autoimmune diseases, perhaps even cancer.

Thus, a clear set of biological mechanisms and processes were documented in laboratory experiments on animals and humans to explain how psychosocial as well as behavioral, environmental, and biomedical risk factors "get under the skin" to cause acute and chronic diseases and sometimes death. Indeed, this evidence showed that the health effects of environmental, behavioral, and psychosocial risk factors for chronic disease often rival or exceed biomedical risk factors.[17]

Historical Epidemiology and Demography and the Impact of Modern Medicine

Finally, in the 1960s, historical epidemiologists and demographers began to reexamine the great decline in mortality and infectious disease between 1750 and 1960. Contrary to the conventional wisdom that the massive improvements in human health and longevity were mainly the product of modern biomedical science and its application via immunization, inoculation, and pharmacologic treatment, these investigations indicated that only a minority of the health improvements over this period—in the range of 20 percent—could plausibly be attributed to modern medical care, as beneficial as that has been. Most seminal and striking was the work of Thomas McKeown, a British professor of social medicine who sought to understand the role of modern biomedical science and practice in the dramatic decline of mortality, especially from infections, in England and Wales in the nineteenth and twentieth centuries.

McKeown focused especially on tuberculosis, which Susan Sontag has termed the cancer of the nineteenth century, accounting for 15 to 20 percent of all deaths in England and Wales at that time. Figure 3.3 shows the steady decline of the death rate from tuberculosis in England and Wales from 1838 until it dropped to close to zero in the 1960s. McKeown pointed out that 50 percent of this decline occurred before Robert Koch discovered the tubercle bacillus in 1882, and also that 80 to 90 percent of the decline took place before effective pharmacologic treatment and vaccination against tuberculosis had been developed in the 1950s. This observation suggested that as little as 10 to 20 percent of the total reduction in tuberculosis mortality from the mid-nineteenth to the mid-twentieth century was attributable to modern biomedical science, and especially its therapeutic or prophylactic application in clinical medicine.[18] Examination of similar U.S. data in the early 1970s showed that the pattern that McKeown observed for tuberculosis (and other infectious diseases) in England and Wales also characterized the United States and most other life-threatening infectious diseases; the exceptions were smallpox, polio (the most recent salient example for people today), and perhaps whooping cough, for all of which vaccination was principally responsible for their decline.[19]

What exactly caused the decline of tuberculosis is more disputed and

Figure 3.3 Respiratory Tuberculosis: Mean Annual Death Rates in England and Wales (Standardized to 1901 Population), 1838–1960

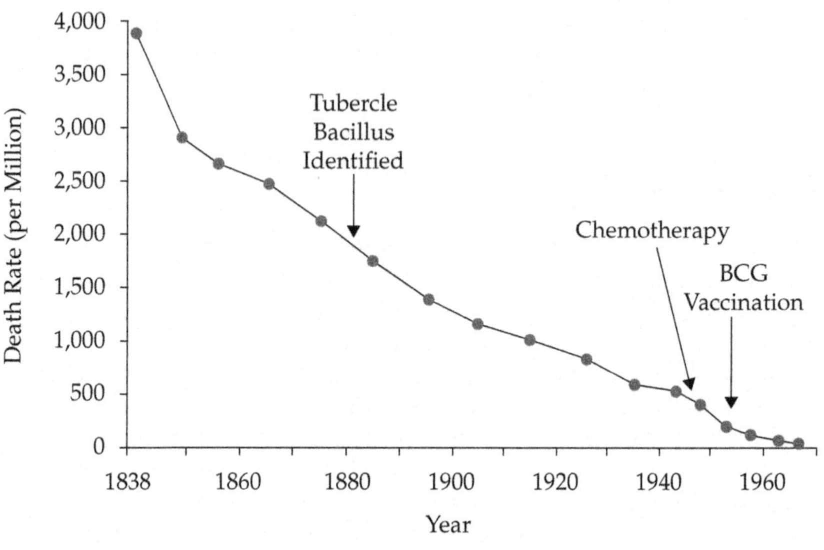

Source: McKeown (1979, figure 8.1). © Princeton University Press (United States, Canada, Philippines, Mexico, and South America) and John Wiley and Sons (all other regions). Reprinted with permission.

harder to establish definitively from historical data. McKeown stressed the role of improved nutrition in increasing host resistance to TB (and other diseases), as many more people are exposed to and even harbor the bacillus than ever succumb to the disease. Other analysts have focused on improvements in all aspects of living conditions—housing and clothing in addition to food—and on general sanitation and public health as also very plausible factors. All of these improvements were made possible by broader social, political, and economic development as well as by the development of biomedical science. All agree, however, that medical care played only a minority role in the dramatic declines in illness and death from infectious disease in Europe and North America in the nineteenth century and the first half of the twentieth century. The major determinants were some combination of social, economic, and environmental factors, and more recent data indicate the same for chronic disease.[20]

McKeown's conclusion that modern biomedical science and practice may have accounted for as little as 10 to 20 percent of the dramatic improvement in life expectancy over the last two hundred to three hundred years has been borne out by other investigators. A careful analysis of the almost thirty-five-year increase in life expectancy in the United States during the twentieth century attributed only about five years (or 15 percent) of that increase to preventive or therapeutic medical care.[21] The vast bulk of this increase seems attributable to a combination of improved sanitation and public health (increasingly informed by modern biomedical science) and, especially, broad patterns of socioeconomic and political development, which enabled improvements in nutrition, clothing, housing, and household sanitation and reductions in the stresses and hazards of long and often dangerous working hours. More recent attempts to estimate the determinants of population health arrive at similar estimates of up to 20 percent for preventive and therapeutic medical care, with the rest attributable to behavioral lifestyle factors (smoking, eating, drinking, and physical activity) and psychosocial and environmental factors.[22]

Unraveling the American Health Paradox: Spending More and Getting Less

Once we recognize that medical care is *not* the major determinant of health, it becomes clearer why spending more and more on increasing the quantity and even the quality of available care does not produce commensurate improvements in the health of individuals and, especially, populations. Indeed, such spending may even be counterproductive to the extent that it diverts resources away from addressing the social, economic, and environmental factors that have a greater role in promoting health and reducing disease.[23] The relation between societal spending on health (which is almost entirely for health care and insurance) and levels of population health is consistent with these conclusions.

Figure 3.4 shows the relation between life expectancy (at birth) and the percentage of GDP spent on health for the twenty-one most-developed Organization for Economic Cooperation and Development (OECD) countries. The correlation (r) is –0.43 overall, and –0.07 if one removes the egregiously outlying case of the United States (an r of 0.00 indicates no relationship and one of 1.00 or –1.00 indicates a perfect positive or negative association, respectively). Thus, all historical and contemporary evidence indicates that increasing societal spending for health care is clearly not the major route to improving population health, and probably never was. And as we will see, spending on a range of other societal goals and services, with which spending on health care and insurance competes, may be the best way to improve health and reduce spending for health care and insurance.

Why Medical Care Is Not More Effective

It must be clearly understood that this is not an indictment of the quality of medical care or its ability to affect and improve health *at the point that it comes into play*. Logically, in fact, we should not expect health care to be the sole or even primary determinant or producer of health, any more

Figure 3.4 Life Expectancy at Birth for Most-Developed OECD Countries by Percentage of GDP Spent on Health, 2006

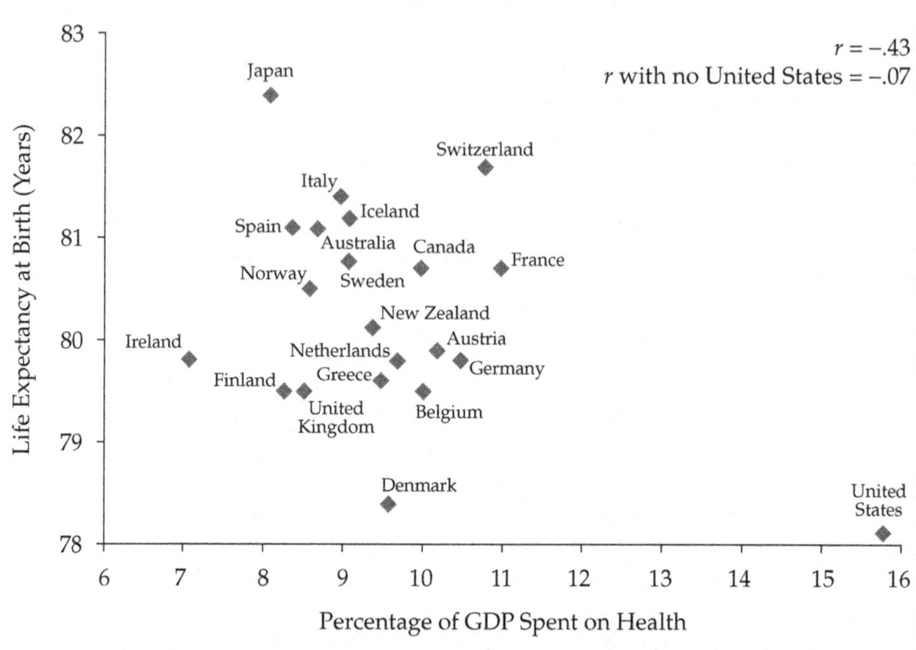

Source: Author compilation based on OECD Factbook (2010) and OECD Health at a Glance (2009).

than we should expect schools to be the sole or perhaps even primary producer of the outcomes we desire from education, considering that children are affected as much or more by what happens in their lives outside of school and before they even start school.

If we think logically about how health and illness are produced, we can readily see that medical care generally comes too little and too late in the process to be more than a minor factor in levels of population health. Figure 3.5 shows the factors that account for the development and onset of any disease, both chronic and acute or infectious, and conversely promote health or resistance to disease. People, like other organisms, are potential hosts to causes of disease because they live in an environment that exposes them to a range of potentially noxious "agents" from viruses and bacteria to environmental pollution and social stresses. They are similarly exposed to salutary agents—from fluoride and nutrients in drinking water and food to benign or supportive physical and social environments—that can promote their resistance as a host to the deleterious effects of potentially noxious agents, or even prevent their exposure to noxious agents in the first place. Individuals are also genetically more

Figure 3.5 Disease Onset as a Function of Environment, Agent, and Host

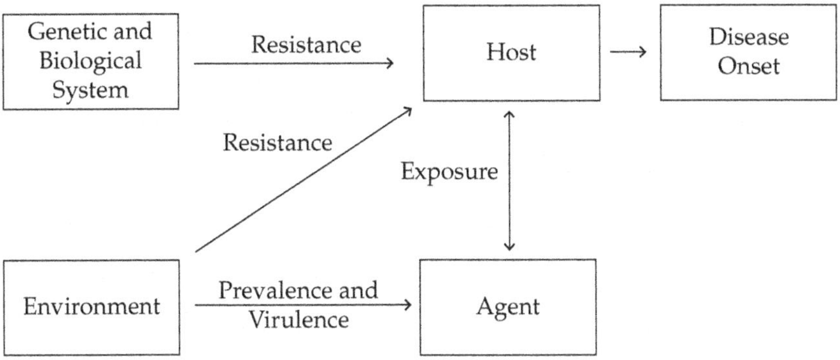

Genetic and Biological System —Resistance→ Host → Disease Onset

Environment —Resistance→ Host

Host ↕ Exposure ↕ Agent

Environment —Prevalence and Virulence→ Agent

Source: Author's compilation.

or less prone or resistant to various diseases, and those tendencies play a significant role in their individual health history. The role of genetics is very small, however, in variations of population health over time and place, because the variation over time and space in the genetic makeup of populations is small.

The medical system generally comes into play only after all of these forces have produced disease in some persons, who then seek treatment. At this point, biomedical science and practice can often take effective, and sometimes quite dramatic, measures to restore health or mitigate the effects of disease. With many chronic diseases, however, the disease process cannot be reversed or eliminated. Rather, it can only be managed more or less well depending on a variety of factors. Clinical practitioners are beginning to recognize this limitation of modern biomedical science. When I ask physicians why they are seeking additional training in the social, psychological, behavioral, and environmental determinants of health, as a growing number of them are doing, they often have the same response: while they and their colleagues can help to improve the health and functioning of the people who appear in their offices and clinics, they recognize that they could do much more by intervening at earlier "upstream" points to prevent the onset, or mitigate the severity, of the chronic and acute injuries and diseases that bring people into the medical system.[24]

At the point when people seek medical care, as indicated in figure 3.6, clinical practitioners are usually trying to manage the further course of disease. Unfortunately, in too many cases, the medical system has little to offer; in others, the recourse is surgical and pharmacological treatments that are quite expensive, have only small to moderate therapeutic effects

Figure 3.6 Medical Care and Disease Onset and Course

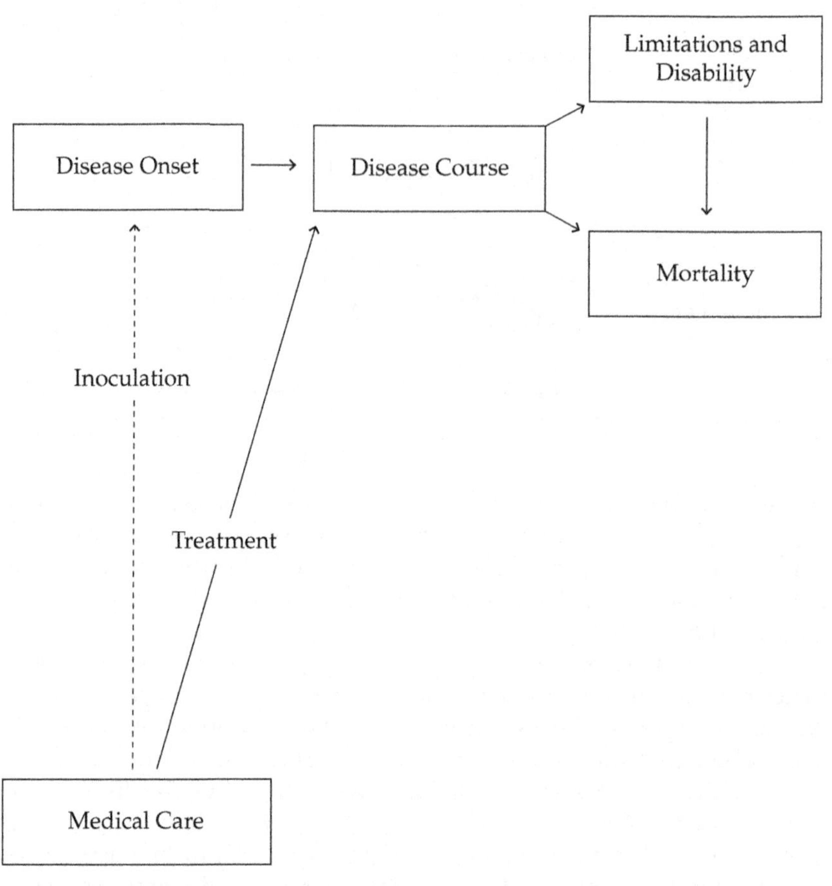

Source: Author's compilation.

on average, and carry nontrivial risks of serious side effects that may be iatrogenic to some extent. For these and other reasons, many practitioners are frustrated by the limits on what they can do, as well as by the societal expectation that they will restore health to people whose life histories and living and working conditions have already overdetermined their downward health trajectory. Further, many practitioners are providing care today with decreasing levels of financial and other supports. If this situation is to change, we need to recall (as indicated in figure 3.7) Virchow's 1848 insight that *broad public policy, including but not limited to or primarily focused on* our current biomedically based health and public

Figure 3.7 Public Policy, Public Health, and Population Health

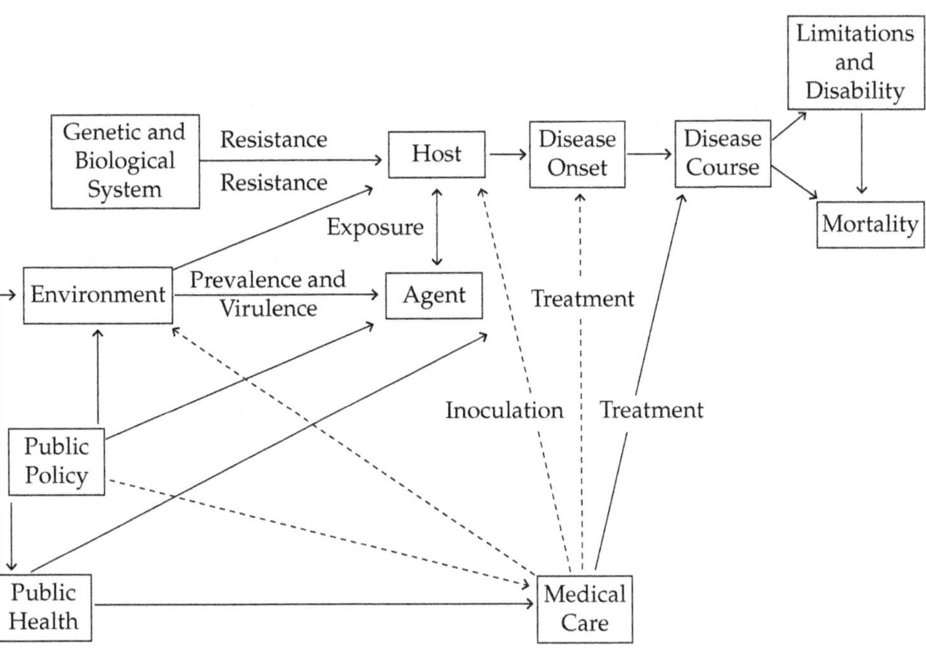

Source: Author's compilation.

health policy, is the ultimate and major determinant of levels of and changes in population health.

To implement such a broad public policy, we need a new demand-side approach to health and health policy that reduces the need to detect and treat disease by focusing much more on creating and sustaining health. In American society, there are both promising and discouraging trends to learn from and to build upon. Chapter 4 provides a framework for thinking about health in a demand-side framework and explores what we know about how and for whom health is currently being most successfully promoted and achieved, and whether and how we might extend these successes to more segments of our society.

Chapter 4

The Lives, Deaths, and Health of Individuals and Populations over Time and Social Strata

ANY DISCUSSION of health science and policy must recognize that health is not like most things that we seek to increase—most noticeably economic ones, which have no inherent limits. In theory at least, there is no cap on how much income or wealth, or how many goods and services, an individual, organization, or society can achieve. Health, in contrast, has real limits established by the evolutionary development of the human organism over millennia. These limits in turn pose some challenges for purely economic ways of thinking about the many major issues in America's paradoxical crisis of health care and health. We can better understand the limits on human health by using sociodemographic approaches at the intersection of sociology, demography, epidemiology, and biomedical science.

Limits on Life and Health over the Life Course of Individuals and Populations

Life and health have clearly finite limits in both individuals and populations. The life span of an individual extends from conception or birth, depending on your perspective, to death. Human evolution has so far resulted in a maximum length to that life span, currently estimated at 110 years on average; the longest known and authenticated length of a human life to date is 122 years. These numbers may not be immutable. But barring a major (and potentially very hazardous) breakthrough that alters the biological and genetic foundations of the human life span, it is likely to continue to grow very gradually at best, notwithstanding the debates in the scientific literature focused as much on fruit flies and rodents as on human beings.[1]

Rectangularization and Compression in Individuals

In light of these current limits on human life span—and for as far ahead as we can reasonably project—the holy grail for individual life and health is to survive in the best possible health for as many of the potential 122 years as possible, until a final brief period of terminal decline. If we visualize our individual life span on a graph, with years of life on the horizontal axis and being alive on the vertical axis, then our life span forms a rectangle, with a line extending across the top for as many years as we live, and then dropping to zero at the moment we die.

Life itself is all or nothing—we are either alive or dead—but our level of health or functioning is not. If we are lucky, we start out at birth in full health—say, at 100 on a scale of 0 to 100. From there—or from a lower point if we are less fortunate—our level of health, as indexed by the absence of morbidity or disease, waxes and wanes, but tending on average to wane with age. Our ability to function physically and mentally is low at birth but generally rises to a peak to which we have evolved in our prime reproductive years, from late adolescence through early adulthood; thereafter, mental and physical functioning also begins to wane. But how early and how rapidly health and functioning wane is highly variable across people. Ideally, our health and functioning would correspond as much as possible to the rectangular distribution of our individual life span. In other words, we are each trying to "rectangularize" or "compress" our levels of health and functioning toward, and ideally almost right up against, the rectangular distribution of our life span. In the best-case scenario, each of us could live to age 122 with good health and functioning and then die over some days, weeks, or months, depending on one's perspective on what constitutes a "good death."

Rectangularization and Compression in Populations

Just as each individual wants to rectangularize and compress her or his mortality, morbidity, and functional limitations or disability, so have human populations sought to do the same. And they have succeeded to a remarkable, if still variable and incomplete, degree. Figures 4.1 and 4.2 graphically depict this aspiration and achievement. Each graph represents on the horizontal axis the years of a human life span from birth (0) to a maximum currently imaginable age of death (125). The vertical axis shows the proportion of a given population age cohort (all people born in a given year) in a given state of health (alive, free of manifest disease or morbidity, or free of functional limitations or disabilities) at each possible year in the human life span.

Figure 4.1 shows how the mortality and life expectancy of human populations has changed over known human history. The far left line

Figure 4.1 The Rectangularization or Compression of Mortality in Human Populations, from More Than 10,000 Years Ago Until the Modern Age

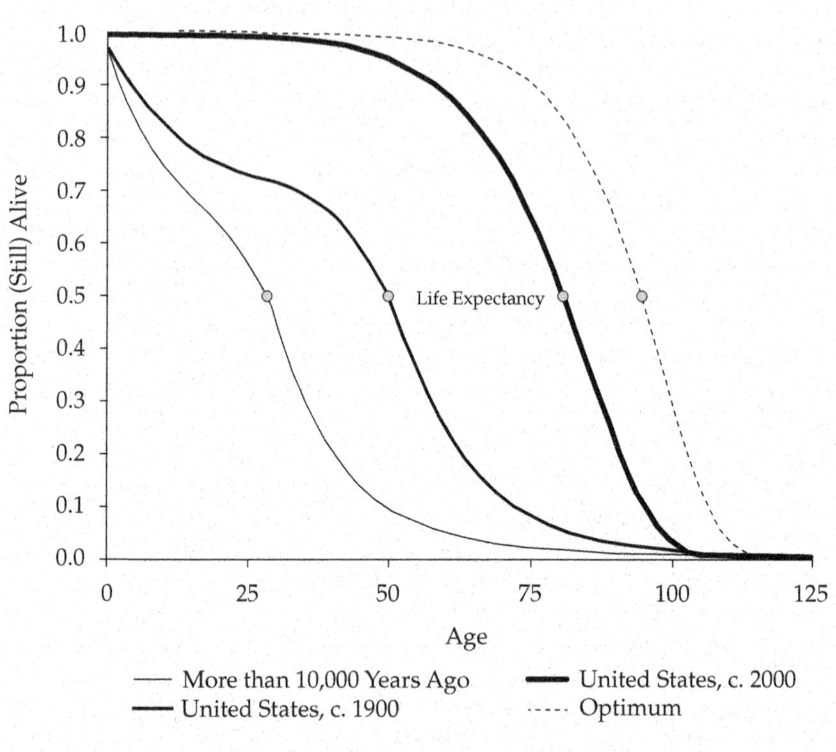

Source: Stylized construction by author (see endnote 4).

shows the situation that characterized all known human populations for millennia up until about 10,000 years ago, when life was still, in the words of the British political philosopher Thomas Hobbes, "nasty, brutish, and short." At that time, and for all prior human history, life expectancy was in the range of twenty-five to thirty years (at which age essentially 50 percent of those born in a given year had died). Thus, a sizable proportion of the population died at birth or in infancy and childhood from disease, malnutrition or starvation, or predation by animals or other humans. The same was true for many of their mothers and fathers by early adulthood, when women also frequently died due to complications of childbirth. Thus, for example, in the population of people born in the year 8000 BC with a life expectancy of twenty-five to thirty years, 50 percent had died by 7070 or 7075 BC. The remainder had better prospects, but continued to have high, age-specific rates of mortality; only a small percentage lived into what we would now call old age.[2]

Mortality began to decline and life expectancy to increase as humans transitioned about 10,000 years ago from nomadic hunting and gathering groups to groups settling in places where they could grow their own food. This communal and agricultural revolution gradually added five to ten years to average human life expectancy, working against the intermittent but often large-scale forces of famine, pestilence, and plague, as well as the downsides of clustering and urbanizing human populations, such as sanitation problems and disease contagion. Thus, even at the beginning of the eighteenth century, average human life expectancy is estimated still to have been only in the range of thirty to thirty-five years.

With the beginning of the industrial revolution in the mid-eighteenth century, human society was rapidly and dramatically transformed in many ways, and none of these changes were more rapid or dramatic than the improvement in human health and longevity. In the 150 or so years from the middle of the eighteenth century to the beginning of the twentieth, life expectancy in the rapidly developing nations of Western Europe and North America increased to almost fifty years (as indicated by the darker line, second from left, in figure 4.1), a greater increase than had occurred in *all* prior human history. In the still shorter period of the twentieth century, life expectancy again increased by more than in all prior human history (including the preceding 150 years of the industrial revolution) to levels approaching or exceeding eighty years in some societies, including the United States (as indicated by the darkest line, third from left, in figure 4.1). This spectacular extension of life expectancy is arguably the greatest single advance in human welfare of all time.

As discussed in chapter 3, the temporal coincidence of the rise of modern biomedicine with this remarkable rise in human health and longevity quite naturally led to the conclusion that modern biomedicine caused the remarkable improvement in human welfare—a conclusion that on closer examination proves illusory, with some grains of truth. Thus, as we concluded in chapter 3, while modern medical care certainly contributed to and helped solidify this remarkable increase of human longevity, it has never been the *primary* cause of increases in human life and health and probably accounts over the last several centuries for only 20 percent or so of the variations in population health and longevity of the now-developed societies.[3]

Unfortunately, neither modern biomedicine nor the socioeconomic, environmental, psychological, and behavioral factors that in combination have been the major causes of past improvements in health and longevity will be able to promote similar rates of improvement in the future. As we have seen in chapter 1 and discussed further in chapter 3, rates of increase in life expectancy in the most-developed countries slowed over the course of the twentieth century: from increases of about twenty years in life span on average over the first half of the twentieth century to about half that number over the second half of the century. The dotted line in figure 4.1 approximates the optimum that the United States and similarly developed societies might achieve in terms of mortality and life expectancy. This possible optimum increase is less than that achieved in the twentieth century alone. Still, there is every reason to believe that in developed nations we will continue to "compress" the mortality and life expectancy distribution of future age cohorts against a biologically limited maximum life span, though perhaps a gradually mutable one. And the overall process is one of increasing rectangularization of the lines graphing these changes, as we observe moving from left to right in figure 4.1.

The be-all and end-all of human life, however, is not its length. We want to live not only a long life but one as free as possible of disease, both infectious and chronic, and of the limitations and disabilities produced by disease and accidental injury. Thus, over time, space, and age cohorts, we seek to "rectangularize" the distribution of these other indicators of health, "compressing" the distribution of these outcomes toward both the biological limits of the human life span and the proximate limits of current life expectancy, as indicated in figure 4.2. The right-hand line in this figure graphs the current mortality and life expectancy curve for the U.S. population; the middle dotted line is the population proportion at different ages without functional limitations or disability; and the proportion without morbidity or disease is the left-hand line. In seeking to rectangularize—or, in other words, to postpone until later ages—the onset of functional limitations, we are essentially trying to compress this curve toward and against the mortality curve. It is less clear whether we can compress the morbidity curve against the functional limitations curve, or to what extent we would want to. Such compression would shorten the years between the onset of disease and functional limitations, but at least in some cases, we may want to diagnose disease earlier so as to better treat or manage it and its functionally limiting sequelae over the long term.[4]

Implications for Health Research and Policy

Several important implications for health research and policy flow from this view of improving individual and population health as a process of rectangularizing and compressing mortality, morbidity, and functional limitations over the life course. First, there are biological limits to how much we can improve health, in all its forms, for any individual or population. Further, individuals and groups in any population vary in how

Figure 4.2 The Rectangularization or Compression of Morbidity and Functional Limitation in U.S. Populations, Circa 2000

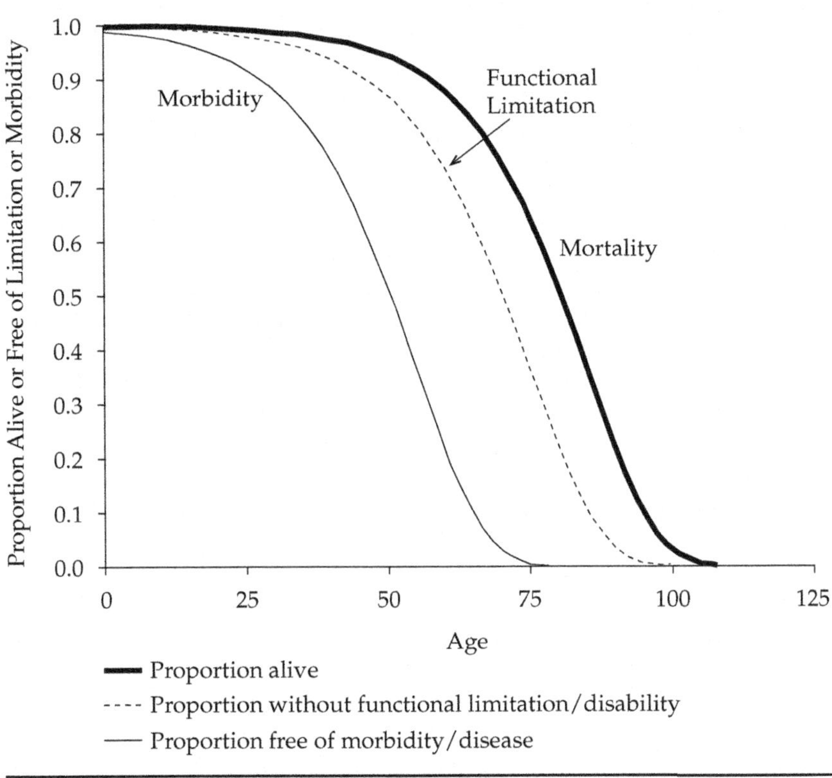

Source: Stylized construction by author (see endnote 4).

close they are to this biological maximum, or optimum. Hence, efforts to further improve health for those close to the biological optimum are likely to have a steeply declining marginal rate of return. In contrast, investments in individuals or groups that are currently furthest from the biological optimum have the highest potential marginal rates of return, not only for improving the health of those individuals and groups but also for improving overall population health.

Second, variations across individuals and population subgroups in life-course trajectories of health are neither random nor genetically fixed. Nor are they primarily a function of medical care, though that is a nontrivial contributing factor. Rather, these variations are mainly driven by varying patterns and conditions of life and work—from health behaviors to psychological dispositions to social and environmental conditions or exposures. Given similar genetic predispositions, people with more favorable conditions of life and work and the associated psychological dispositions and behavioral lifestyles that promote or protect health are more likely to approach the optimal or maximal trajectories of health over the life course. To the extent that we can not only improve accessibility to and utilization of medical care among the less healthy but also make their conditions of life and work closer to conditions for healthier people, we should see the life-course patterns of mortality, morbidity, and limitations and disability among the less healthy begin to approximate those of the healthier.

Finally, conditions of life and work do not vary randomly or independently of each other. Rather, they cluster within individuals and social groups—among whom some have relatively positive profiles on all or most of these conditions, while others have profiles that are more adverse or risky for health. Understanding how and why such clustering occurs is key to moving those with adverse or risky conditions of life and work toward more favorable conditions, and hence improving their health trajectories over the life course. In the rest of this chapter and the next one, we will examine the crucial role of several key bases of social differentiation and inequality—socioeconomic position, race-ethnicity, and gender—in the clustering of both risky and protective factors for health in the United States and, to varying degrees, in other societies.

Both health research and health policy have given the implications of biological limits on health insufficient recognition and emphasis. One important implication is that the rates of return from increasing our investments in producing and improving health must sooner or later begin to diminish, sooner for some individuals or portions of the population and later for others. As we approach the biological limits on health—as individuals, groups, or whole societies—we must be sensitive to these changing rates of return and become more strategic in making investments that go toward the people and population groups for whom the potential for improving health over the life course remains substantial.

Health research and policy must also identify more broadly the kinds of investments that have the greatest returns to population health—what a Virchow of today might term "comparative effectiveness research on a grand scale." This shift in focus would consider not only biomedical health care and insurance policy but also all conditions of life and work, and thus all aspects of public policy.[5] Finally, and perhaps most importantly, health research and health policy need to focus much more on identifying disparities across individuals and populations in the degree to which their health across the life span is rectangularized and compressed. Addressing these disparities is not only a matter of social justice, important as that is, but also the key to taking the most cost-effective approach to sustaining and improving levels of mortality, morbidity, and functional limitation in the U.S. population and in other human populations.

The (Re)Discovery of Socioeconomic Disparities in Health

The Lack of Awareness in the Late Nineteenth Century to the Mid-Twentieth Century

Although Virchow and others had observed major socioeconomic differences in health in the mid-nineteenth century, attention to and serious investigation of such differences declined from the late nineteenth century through the mid-twentieth century, just as Emil Behring had argued that it should in 1893 (see chapter 3). With the major focus of biomedicine on controlling infectious diseases via vaccines and pharmaceuticals derived from bacteriologic and virologic science, little consideration was given to broader social and environmental factors (except for efforts to eliminate infectious agents from any and all environments). Because infectious disease could strike persons from all walks of life, some historical analysts have argued that socioeconomic differences in morbidity and mortality from infectious disease were small or nonexistent in many populations as late as the end of the nineteenth and early twentieth centuries.[6]

In the decades immediately after World War II, these potential reasons for ignoring socioeconomic and racial-ethnic disparities were reinforced by a growing belief that new economic and political developments and policies were drastically reducing or eliminating abject poverty and deprivation and more generally muting economic, or "class," and racial-ethnic differences. These developments included economic growth that "lifted all boats," civil rights and social welfare policies that reduced racial-ethnic, gender, and socioeconomic inequalities, and public health care and insurance policies that by 1970 provided universal access to modern medical care in almost all highly developed countries. Even the laggard and exceptional United States was providing universal coverage for the elderly and many of the poor via Medicare and Medicaid and covering most workers in larger firms and their families under a steadily growing employer-based health insurance system.

Even the scientific discipline most focused on social inequalities showed little concern about social disparities in health. In 1972 the editors of the second edition of the *Handbook of Medical Sociology* noted, with a combination of surprise and embarrassment, "As remarkable as it may seem, neither the terms 'poverty' nor 'Negro,' let alone 'black,' were employed frequently enough by contributors [to the first *Handbook of Medical Sociology* of 1963] for the editors to include them in the Index!"[7]

Late Twentieth-Century (Re)Discovery: The Black Report and Its Impact

Disregard and complacency regarding socioeconomic and other social inequalities in health was starkly challenged in 1980 in the United Kingdom by the "Report of the Working Group on Inequalities in Health," since known as the "Black Report," after the chair of the working group, Sir Douglas Black, the British equivalent of the Surgeon General of the United States. The Black Report ultimately had a scientific and political impact as great or greater than the Surgeon General's report on smoking and health in 1964, but not the same policy impact owing to the political circumstances under which it was commissioned and delivered, as well as its politically charged findings and recommendations.

The Labor government of Prime Minister James Callaghan had commissioned the working group in the late 1970s, but by the time it delivered its report in 1980 the Conservatives, under Margaret Thatcher, had come to power. Their response via the Secretary of State for Social Services, Patrick Jenkins, was to acknowledge the receipt of the Black Report with perfunctory thanks and to dismiss its policy recommendations while questioning its scientific quality and conclusions via faint praise:

> The Working Group on Inequalities in Health was set up in 1977, on the initiative of my predecessor as Secretary of State, under the Chairmanship of Sir Douglas Black, to review information about differences in health status between the social classes; to consider possible causes and the implications for policy; and to suggest further research.
>
> The Group was given a formidable task, and Sir Douglas and his colleagues deserve thanks for seeing the work through, and for the thoroughness with which they have surveyed the considerable literature on the subject. As they make clear, the influences at work in explaining the relative health experience of different parts of our society are many and interrelated; and, while it is disappointing that the Group were unable to make greater progress in disentangling the various causes of inequalities in health, the difficulties they experienced are perhaps no surprise given current measurement techniques.
>
> It will come as a disappointment to many that over long periods since the inception of the NHS there is generally little sign of health inequalities in Britain actually diminishing and, in some cases, they may be increasing. It will be seen that the Group has reached the view that the causes of health inequalities are so deep rooted that only a major and wide-ranging pro-

> gramme of public expenditure is capable of altering the pattern. I must make it clear that additional expenditure on the scale which could result from the report's recommendations—the amount involved could be upwards of £2 billion a year—is quite unrealistic in present or any foreseeable economic circumstances, quite apart from any judgement that may be formed of the effectiveness of such expenditure in dealing with the problems identified. I cannot, therefore, endorse the Group's recommendations. I am making the report available for discussion, but without any commitment by the Government to its proposals.[8]

The Black Report showed, most importantly, that over a quarter-century of operation the National Health Service had not diminished the absolute or relative differences in mortality rates by social (actually occupational) class and that, as even Patrick Jenkins conceded, "in some cases" they may have been increasing more rapidly in the two decades after 1950 than before then. The report thoroughly documented these trends and thoughtfully explored the reasons for them, if not to the satisfaction of Mr. Jenkins or Mrs. Thatcher.

Only 250 duplicated copies of the report were made available on the 1980 August bank holiday when it was released. However, a "slightly slimmed down version" was republished in 1982 by Penguin Press.[9] Widely read and discussed, the Black Report ultimately led to socioeconomic and other social disparities in health becoming the leading foci of social epidemiologic research and public health policy in many countries, including the United States.

U.S. Department of Health and Human Services scientists found similar results for educational differences in mortality among working-age (twenty to sixty-six) adults between 1960 and 1986, as shown in figure 4.3.[10] Although death rates declined for everyone, they declined more rapidly among the highly educated. Consequently, for men, the differences in *absolute* death rates between those with low versus high education grew from about four per thousand (ten versus six) in 1960 to about five per thousand (eight versus three) in 1986, and *relative* differences (the ratio of the low-educated rate to the high-educated rate in each year) grew from about 1.7:1 to 2.7:1. Female educational differences in death rates were smaller in that period, but also grew absolutely and relatively, and since 1986 they have increasingly come to approach the educational differences in men. Analyses in Canada found much the same, even after a quarter-century of national health insurance.[11]

A Personal Epiphany

My colleagues and I also rediscovered the extent and importance of socioeconomic differences in health soon after launching in 1986 a national

Figure 4.3 Death Rates Among U.S. Whites Age Twenty-Five to Sixty-Four, by Sex and Educational Level, 1960 and 1986

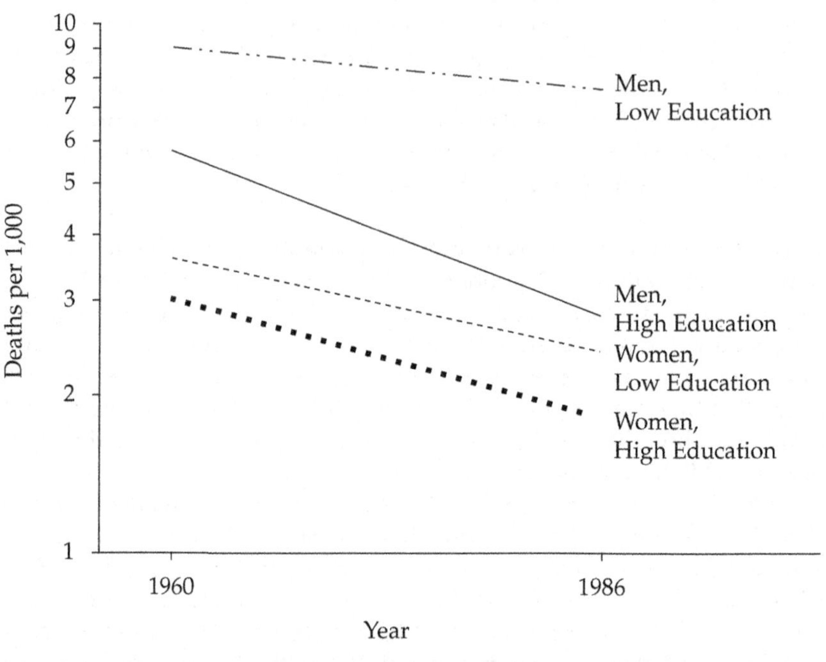

Source: Pappas et al. (1994, figure 4). © 1993 Massachusetts Medical Society. Reprinted with permission.

longitudinal, or prospective, study of the role of social, psychological, and behavioral factors in the maintenance of health and effective functioning over the adult life course. The study, which we named the Americans' Changing Lives (ACL) study, began with a nationally representative (excluding Alaska and Hawaii) survey of 3,617 adults age twenty-five and older. We reinterviewed survivors in 1989, 1994, 2001–2002, and late 2011–early 2012, as described more fully in box 4.1.

When the 1986 survey became ready for analysis, we initially sought to explore the factors that contributed most to the maintenance of health and effective functioning over the life course. We examined how measures of health varied by age for different subgroups of the population, such as men versus women, blacks versus whites, smokers versus nonsmokers, socially isolated versus socially integrated, and higher versus lower education or income. The strongest predictors by far of successful health maintenance (rectangularization and compression) and effective functioning over the life course were two indicators of socioeconomic position: education and income.

Box 4.1 Timeline for the Americans' Changing Lives (ACL) Study

1986: Nationally representative cross-section survey of the U.S. population age twenty-five and older

- Oversampling of blacks (2:1) and persons age sixty and older (2:1)
- Sample size = 3,617
- Response rate = 68 to 70 percent
- Eighty-six-minute face-to-face interview

1989: Eighty-nine-minute face-to-face reinterviews of 2,867 survivors (83 percent)

1994: Forty-five-minute telephone or face-to-face reinterviews of 2,559 survivors (83 percent)

2001–2002: Forty-five-minute telephone or face-to-face reinterviews of 1,785 survivors (74 percent)

2011–2012: Seventy-minute telephone or face-to-face reinterviews of 1,427 survivors (81 percent)

1986–2011: Continuous mortality tracking via the National Death Index and other methods

From the beginning, we chose to focus on a measure of functional limitations, since that was the single most valid and reliable way to measure health in our self-report interviews. (Since 1986, we have also tracked the mortality of our respondents.) We asked respondents how much difficulty they had in doing a range of activities, from getting out of bed or a chair and using the toilet to walking a few blocks or up a few flights of stairs, to doing heavy work around the house like shoveling snow or washing walls. We used respondents' reports that they could do any and all of these things, even shoveling snow or washing walls, with little or no difficulty as the single most reliable indicator of health.

Figure 4.4 graphs the proportion of respondents at three levels of education who reported no functional limitations (vertical axis) by their age when interviewed in 1986 (horizontal axis). Viewed in the rectangularization and compression framework, we see substantial differences by education: those with the lowest education (less than high school—the line with triangles) manifested almost no rectangularization or compression; rather, they showed an almost linear decline in functional health

Figure 4.4 Functional Limitations of U.S. Adults from Early Adulthood to Late Old Age, by Education: ACL Study, 1986

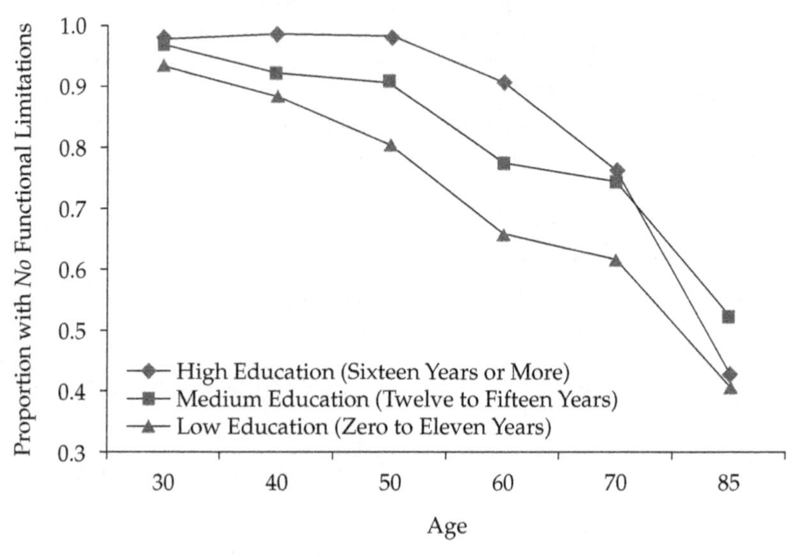

Source: Adapted from House et al. (1994, figure 1).

from early adulthood (age twenty-five to thirty-four) through later old age (eighty and older). In contrast, the most highly educated (college graduates or higher—the line with diamonds) manifested notable rectangularization and compression: they remained almost entirely free of limitations through their midfifties, then began to decline at increasingly greater rates over the remainder of the life course. The middle educational group (high school graduates with up to some college education—the line with squares) generally lay between these two groups.

Viewed another way, these data suggest that educational disparities in functional limitations vary over the life course, being small in early adulthood (the reproductive and child-rearing years, during which we have evolved to be at our most robust), increasingly larger over the adult working years, then smaller again as we become biologically frailer with age, until, in the words of John Maynard Keynes, "in the long run we all are dead."[12]

We and others have observed similar patterns of results for mortality, morbidity, and other measures of functional limitations. And we have seen similar patterns by income, though further analysis has suggested that education is more important in postponing the onset of health problems, while income is more important in slowing the progression of health problems once they occur, up to and including death.[13]

What is most notable in figure 4.4 (and in similar graphs by income or for morbidity and mortality outcomes) is the size of the socioeconomic differences in functional health—which reach absolute differences of twenty-five to thirty percentage points at their peak between ages fifty-five and sixty-five. Viewed in terms of rectangularization and compression of functional limitation, these are *differences of twenty-five to thirty years on average in the rate of aging in terms of functional limitation:* people in the lowest socioeconomic groups manifest levels of functional limitations by age thirty-four to forty-four that are not seen in the highest socioeconomic groups until ages fifty-five to sixty-four (in the case of education) or sixty-five to seventy-four (in the case of income). A qualitative researcher, Katherine Newman, once remarked to me that she sees these differences in the faces of her respondents. For example, many of her disadvantaged respondents whom she knows to be age forty-five or younger look like they are seventy. We have all seen the same in people who we say "have had a hard life"—which is exactly the reason they are prematurely aged and less healthy than their more fortunate age peers.[14]

Why Are Socioeconomic Disparities in Health So Large?

The $64,000 question remains: why are there such large health disparities by education and other socioeconomic variables such as income, occupation, and wealth?[15] A variety of evidence indicates that there are some socioeconomic differences in access to and utilization of medical care. However, for reasons discussed in chapters 2 and 3, neither these differences nor the relationship between medical care and health are anywhere near strong enough to explain the socioeconomic disparities in levels and trajectories of health over the life course that have been observed. A more plausible hypothesis is that these disparities are explained by the greater exposure of those at lower socioeconomic levels to a broad range of the social, psychological, behavioral, environmental, and biomedical risk factors for health discussed in chapter 3.

A Conceptual Framework for Understanding Social Inequalities in Health and Aging

Figure 4.5 graphically depicts this broad hypothesis, which is based on more general social science understanding of education and income, as well as on other aspects of socioeconomic position, such as occupation and wealth as basic resources that determine people's ability to achieve more desirable conditions of life and work, including conditions that affect health. What makes these socioeconomic variables so powerful is that they shape people's experiences of and exposure to *any and all* health

Figure 4.5 A Conceptual Framework for Understanding Social Inequalities in Health and Aging

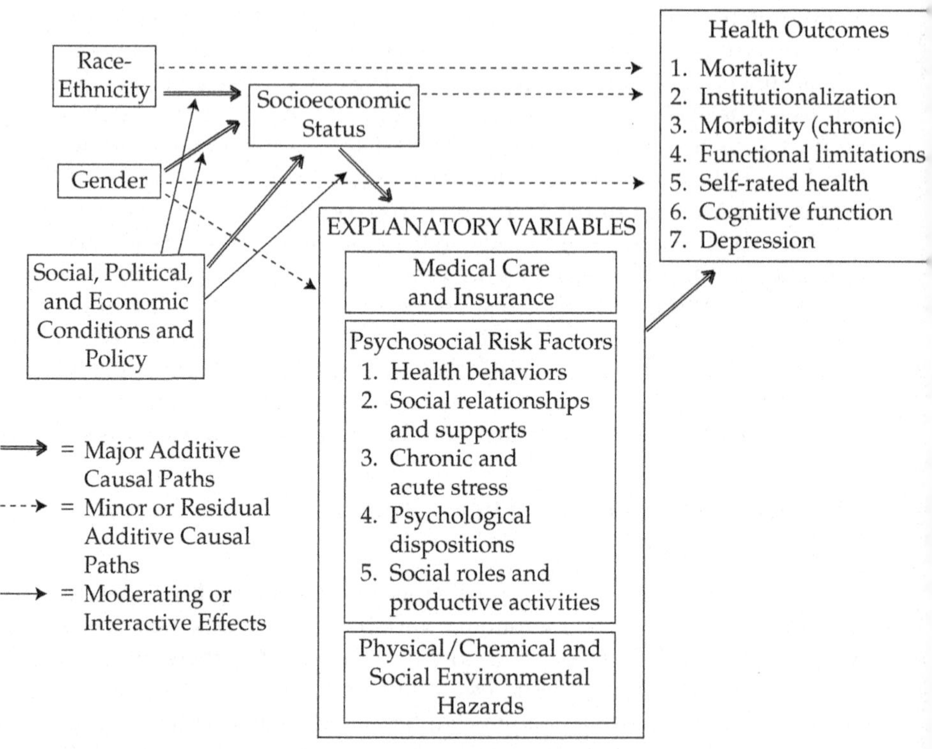

Source: Adapted from House (2002, figure 5).

risk factors and continue to do so even as the major diseases that cause health problems and the causal risk factors for them change over time.

We have seen historically that, at least since the early twentieth century, as a disease has emerged and increased in importance as a source of mortality or functional limitations and disability, it has developed an inverse relation with indicators of socioeconomic position. For example, at the beginning of the twentieth century, coronary heart disease was as common at upper socioeconomic levels as at lower ones, if not more so. By midcentury this relationship began to reverse, and by the end of the twentieth century heart disease, like most other major diseases, had become more common at lower socioeconomic levels than at upper ones. Similarly, major risk factors for heart disease and cancer, such as smoking cigarettes, eating a high-fat diet, or having a sedentary lifestyle (and hence problems like obesity), were more common at higher socioeconomic levels when they first emerged in the late nineteenth and early twentieth centuries. But again, over the course of the twentieth century these risk factors became much more characteristic of persons at lower socioeconomic levels. And even a totally new disease such as AIDS, which first emerged in socioeconomically advantaged portions of the population, rapidly became more incident and prevalent among persons of lower socioeconomic position (and of nonwhite racial-ethnic status). For these reasons, socioeconomic position has aptly been described by Bruce Link and Jo Phelan as a "fundamental cause" of disease and ill health.[16]

Evidence for the Framework

If socioeconomic position has been and remains such a fundamental cause of ill health, we expected that any and eventually almost all risk factors for health would be more prevalent at lower socioeconomic levels. This seemed to be the case in the broader scientific literature that we knew, but we also sought to determine the extent to which this was the case in our ACL data. The results were as expected—and distressing beyond even our direst expectations. We found that almost all psychosocial and behavioral risk factors for health in our data were more prevalent at lower socioeconomic levels, even ones that have become economically costly, such as smoking. As had others, we observed that people of lower education and income were more likely to smoke, to be sedentary outside of work, and to eat or drink immoderately.[17] In addition, we also found a whole range of psychosocial risk factors for health. Each of these risk factors has been shown in prospective studies to predict mortality, morbidity, and functional problems and disability, but they had not all been previously measured in a single national study that showed them to be much more prevalent at lower educational (figure 4.6) and income (figure 4.7) levels.

Figures 4.6 and 4.7 include a wide range of psychosocial risk factors: social isolation or lack of relationships (being unmarried, never attending meetings of clubs and organizations, and talking with others less than once a week in person or by phone), psychological states or dispositions known to be risky for health (high hostility, a low sense of self-efficacy, control, or mastery, and depressive symptoms), and stress (a count of negative life events such as widowhood, divorce, or unemployment). In all cases, these psychosocial risk factors are anywhere from *one and a half to almost five times more prevalent at lower levels of education and income* (except for the relation of negative life events with education, which shows only a small and not statistically significant difference). Similarly, in all but two cases (depressive symptoms and negative life events by education), there is a clear and consistent gradient from lower to higher education and income.

Figure 4.6 Psychosocial Risk Factor Status in U.S. Residents Age Forty-Five to Sixty-Four, by Education: ACL Study, 1986

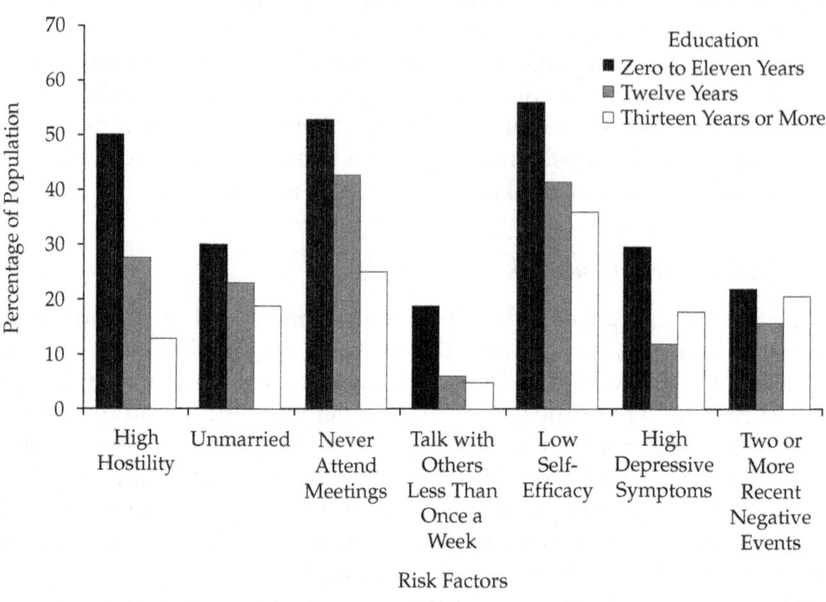

Sources: House and Williams (2000, figure 2A). For hostility: Minnesota Multiphasic Personality Inventory (MMPI) Standardization Study.

If it is exposure to these risk factors and others that explains the poorer health and life-course health trajectories of those in lower socioeconomic strata, then socioeconomic disparities should be greatly reduced if lower and higher socioeconomic strata were not to differ on such experiences and exposures. And this is exactly what we found, as shown in figure 4.8. The solid lines in figure 4.8 merely reproduce figure 4.4, and the dotted lines show what happens when we statistically adjust for a set of eleven psychosocial risk factors (including health behaviors, acute and chronic stress, social relationships, and psychological status or disposition) as well as income (which is heavily a function of education and was increasingly so over the course of the twentieth century). The dotted lines show that statistically equalizing the experience of and exposure to these risks across educational groups eliminates 80 to 90 percent of the twenty- to thirty-percentage-point educational disparities in freedom from functional limitations that we observed in figure 4.4 for the peak working years of the adult life course. That is, if lower-educated people had the same income and risk factor experience and exposure as the higher-educated, they would manifest levels of health and rectangularization and compression similar to levels for the higher-educated. About half of

Figure 4.7 Psychosocial Risk Factor Status in U.S. Residents Age Forty-Five to Sixty-Four, by Income: ACL Study, 1986

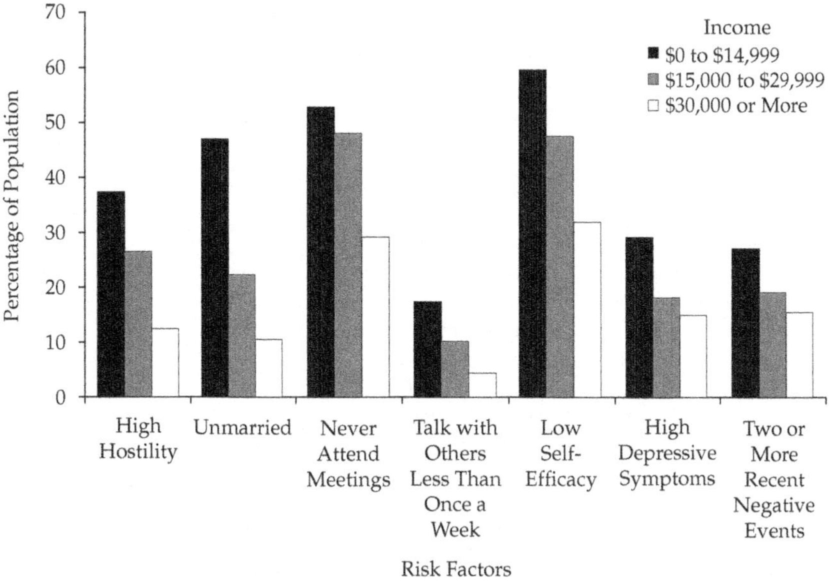

Sources: House and Williams (2000, figure 2B). For hostility: MMPI Standardization Study.

the explanatory power comes from the better incomes earned by more-educated people and about half from the psychosocial and behavioral risk factors.[18]

Relationships in figures 4.4 and 4.6 to 4.8 derive from cross-sectional (1986) data and thus are subject to concerns over the direction of causality. (Does socioeconomic position cause health, or vice versa?) Our early data also did not allow enough time to observe major changes in health, including substantial numbers of deaths. To compensate for the causal ambiguities we increasingly have focused on levels of education, which are determined and fixed relatively early in adult life and thus cannot be affected by later health.

Further Longitudinal Analysis

To further minimize these causal ambiguities and observe greater changes in health within individuals we extended the follow-up of our ACL survey through 1989 to 1994, 2001–2002, and now 2011–2012. The data through 1994 clearly established that both education and income as assessed in 1986 predicted mortality in the ACL sample between 1986 and

Figure 4.8 Functional Limitations of U.S. Adults from Early Adulthood to Late Old Age, by Education, Before and After Adjustment for Income and Eleven Psychosocial Risk Factors: ACL Study, 1986

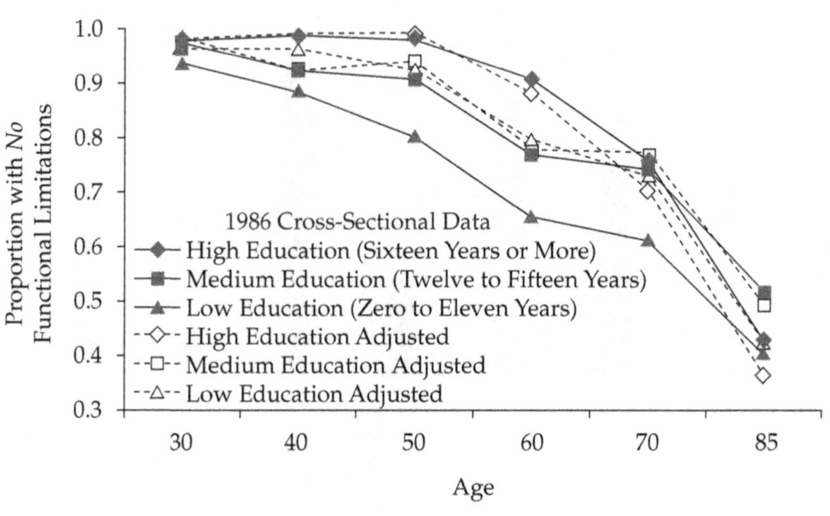

Source: Adapted from House et al. (1994, figure 3).

1994. The mortality risk of low education or low income proved much greater than the risk of any other single risk factor (for example, smoking). Consistent with our earlier findings, and with the cross-sectional, longitudinal, and prospective findings of others, socioeconomic disparities in health and the way health changes with age cannot be explained by any single risk factor or by a small set of risk factors. Even measures of a broad domain, like health behaviors (as indexed by smoking, drinking, weight or obesity, and physical activity) or stress (including both life events and chronic stress), can usually account for no more than 15 to 30 percent of the educational or income disparities in health. Our research and especially the research of others suggest that the same is true of medical care and insurance: that is, it is the greater experience of or exposure to virtually *all* health risk factors among people of lower socioeconomic position (as in figures 4.6, 4.7, and 4.8) that accounts for their lower levels of health and poorer life-course trajectories.[19]

In cross-sectional data, disparities in health and in the ways health changes with age appear quite similar by education and income. However, educational and income disparities manifest somewhat different properties and processes over time. In our data and that of others, education seems especially important in postponing the onset of health problems, while income is more important, both absolutely and relative to education, in predicting the course of health among those with health problems up to and including death. This reflects both education's continuous effect over the life course and the resources that education provides for understanding and utilizing preventive health behaviors and health care. In contrast, income provides resources that can be brought to bear in adapting to or alleviating the course of illness. Higher-income people are better able to pay for medical care, to retire sooner, to move to healthier environments and improve their living conditions, and to acquire and use assistive technology to maintain functioning.[20]

Whither Social Disparities in Rectangularization/Compression of Health: Empirical and Conceptual Issues

The last few centuries have brought dramatic rectangularization and compression of mortality toward the biological limits of the human life span, as well as rectangularization and compression of morbidity and functional limitations toward the current levels of life expectancy. Less clear is how well we are succeeding in rectangularizing and compressing morbidity and functional limitations relative to the rectangularization and compression of mortality. When we began our ACL study in 1986, it was hotly contested whether advances in life expectancy were not simply "adding years to life," but also "life to years." Or, in a more pessimistic phrasing, were we simply achieving "longer life, but worse health"? Were we more rapidly adding years of life with significant morbidity and disability than adding years of life with good health and little or no limitation or disability?[21]

In the early 1970s through the early 1980s, it looked like the pessimists were closer to the truth. By the later 1980s and early 1990s, however, the evidence suggested that disability levels were beginning to decline in the elderly population.[22] This suggested to at least some analysts that even if the United States was not doing as well as other countries in overall population health, we might have been doing as well as others for the elderly, or even better.[23] Like the larger fields of public health, medical sociology, and social gerontology, however, this debate largely failed to take account of social disparities in health and the ways in which health changes with age.

Our figure 4.4 and other data suggest that the positive gains were very likely occurring only or mainly for the advantaged parts of the population.[24] Thus, growing social disparities in health arose as people aged through middle and early old age, with such disparities gradually diminishing as everyone became frailer in later stages of old age (see figure 4.4). It therefore became important to us to understand whether reductions in older-age disability in the later 1980s and 1990s were continuing into the twenty-first century, and if so, whether they were doing so in ways that would maintain, enhance, or reduce social disparities in health over the life course.

Data from reinterviews with our ACL sample in 2001–2002, fifteen years after we first interviewed them in 1986, showed similar evidence of decline in functional limitations at older ages, especially among the highly educated, but otherwise little change from the pattern of change in functional limitations by levels of age and education seen in figure 4.4.

Several important conclusions emerge from comparing the changes in functional limitations for people of different ages and education between 1986 and 2001–2002 to the cross-sectional snapshot as of 1986 seen in figure 4.4. First, the cross-sectional differences in health at different ages in 1986 are not simply the residues of the education differences in health produced earlier in life and carried forward as people age, but rather reflections of the way health changes as people age. Second, the one exception to the pattern of overlap between the cross-sectional and longitudinal results occurred for people of higher education: only 60 percent of college-educated people age seventy to eighty-four in 1986 were free of functional limitations, whereas by 2001–2002 almost 85 percent of the college-educated of this age reported no functional limitations. Indeed, college-educated people who were fifty-five to sixty-nine in 1986 experienced virtually no changes in functional limitation as they aged to become seventy to eighty-four in 2001–2002—hence greatly increasing the rectangularization and compression of their functional limitations into later old age.

Unfortunately, people who were comparably aged (fifty-five to sixty-nine) in 1986 and had lower levels of education showed no evidence of such improvements. As a result, *educational disparities in functioning in older age* (seventy to eighty-four) *were four times greater by 2001–2002 than they had been in 1986* (forty percentage points versus ten percentage points, respectively).[25]

Thus, the last ten to fifteen years of the twentieth century were characterized by some improvements in population health in late middle through early to middle old age, mainly and perhaps only at higher educational levels. These improvements increased socioeconomic disparities in health and extended them further into older age. The hope was that gains at higher levels of education might extend even later in the life course and come over time to be replicated at lower socioeconomic levels, further improving overall population health and reducing social disparities in health.

Unfortunately, data from the end of the first decade of the twenty-first century indicate that disability is no longer declining at older ages. Initial analyses of the fifth wave of our ACL data collected in 2011–2012 are consistent with these results. In the first decade of the twenty-first century, we observe no evidence or further extensions of the rectangularization and compression of functional limitations among the highly educated (age seventy to eighty-four in 2001–2002). More distressingly, we see no evidence that those age fifty-five to sixty-nine in 2001–2002 are even repeating the gains that those of that age in 1986 made as they aged to become seventy to eighty-four.[26] Nor has anything improved for lower socioeconomic levels.

Socioeconomic Disparities in Health and Health Policy

Early in the second decade of the twenty-first century, the United States is characterized by large, persistent, and probably increasing socioeconomic disparities in health. These disparities are generally larger than those in comparably developed nations.[27] Although levels of life expectancy continue to improve, it is not clear that these increased years of life are accompanied by reductions in functional limitations and disability at older ages, even at higher socioeconomic levels.

Still the higher socioeconomic strata are now doing almost as well as any populations in the world—and increasingly as well as is biologically possible. Hence, the major need and opportunity for improving the health of the American population lies in improving the health of the lower socioeconomic strata. Reducing social disparities in health is not just a matter of social justice but also the most cost-effective path to improving overall population health and hence reducing the need for health care utilization and expenditure, both absolutely and relative to other nations. Reducing social disparities in health could also resolve America's paradoxical crisis of health care and health, or go a long way toward doing so.

The challenge is to extend the improvements in health that have been made in the upper socioeconomic strata to the lower socioeconomic levels. This will require improving the income levels of lower socioeconomic people, and perhaps especially their educational level, as well as helping them gain access to the resources and benefits that have enabled dramatic advances in health at higher income and educational levels: health-promoting behaviors, greater access to and utilization of health care, and better conditions of life and work.

We know that socioeconomic position shapes the experience of and exposure to virtually all social, psychological, behavioral, environmental, and biomedical risk factors for health. And it similarly shapes resources for adapting to problems in life, work, and health. Fundamental cause theory argues for a focus on the socioeconomic factors that tend to drive variation in all risk factors for health, but progress can also be made by identifying and focusing on key social, psychological, behavioral, and environmental factors, such as social isolation, depression, smoking, and air pollution. Before we turn to look at how health research and policy might move toward these goals, we need to recognize that health and social disparities in health are driven not only by socioeconomic factors but also by the sociobiological factors of race-ethnicity, gender, and age—even if, as we will see, socioeconomic factors account for some, even many, of the variations and disparities in health along these dimensions.

Chapter 5

Racial-Ethnic, Gender, and Age Disparities in Health and Their Relation to Socioeconomic Position

Social disparities in health are not just socioeconomic. They also occur by race-ethnicity, gender, and even age. Indeed, in the popular mind, and perhaps even more in political and governmental arenas, the term "social disparities in health" is as likely to connote racial-ethnic, gender, or age disparities as socioeconomic ones, if not more so. For example, the newest institute of the National Institutes of Health (NIH), charged with doing research and training on social disparities in health, is the National Institute of Minority Health and Health Disparities, which prioritizes, at least in name, racial-ethnic disparities in health. Since 1991, NIH has also had a Women's Health Initiative to improve epidemiologic understanding and clinical treatment of women's health, particularly postmenopausal health. Nowhere in NIH is there a unit or program focused on socioeconomic disparities in health, although these are addressed in many centers and institutes.

This all reflects a broader approach to social disparities and inequalities in America. The Constitution and related legislative, executive, and judicial actions specifically proscribe discrimination or unfair treatment on the basis of race-ethnicity, sex-gender, and age, but not on the basis of any aspect of socioeconomic position. The assumption is that race-ethnicity, sex-gender, and age are, in sociological terminology, "ascribed" statuses—essentially determined or given at birth. In contrast, socioeconomic positions or statuses are conceived as "achieved," the outcome of individual effort and behavior, albeit in the context of complex and often constraining social systems of education and work. Differences across ascribed statuses in the attainments and situations of people, including their health, are hence assumed to reflect potential discrimination or unfair treatment, but no such assumption is made regarding differences in socioeconomic attainments.

Racial-ethnic, gender, and age disparities in health are also large. This is obvious for age, where the issue is to recognize that some of these differences are due to psychosocial factors and not just to biological ones. Basic gender differences are also well known: women live longer than men in almost all societies, currently by about five years in the United States; yet women are more likely to suffer from a number of prevalent chronic diseases and disabilities. Racial differences are large and longstanding: whites on average currently live almost five years longer than blacks, with almost seven years' difference among men. These racial and gender differences cumulate, so that white women now live about ten years longer than black men, with life expectancies of eighty-one and seventy-one, respectively.[1]

Socioeconomic disparities in life expectancy, however, and in health more generally, tend to be even larger than either racial-ethnic or gender disparities. Moreover, racial-ethnic and gender disparities are also partially explained by differences in socioeconomic position. And like socioeconomic disparities, racial-ethnic, gender, and even some age disparities in health are explainable in terms of differential exposure to and experience of a wide range of social, environmental, psychological, and behavioral risk factors for health, even as potential and actual biological factors are taken into account. Thus, I have prioritized socioeconomic factors in discussing social disparities in health.

Racial-ethnic, gender, and age differences and disparities in health could each receive book-length treatment. Here I want to clarify three issues with respect to these three areas: (1) the degree to which each reflects biological versus other factors; (2) the degree to which nonbiological differences or disparities are a function of socioeconomic factors; and (3) the extent to which other nonbiological factors are involved. Overall, we will see that racial-ethnic, gender, and age disparities in health can largely be explained in the same ways as socioeconomic ones, and also in varying degrees *by* socioeconomic disparities. The remainder of this chapter considers racial-ethnic, gender, and age disparities in health in order of the relative role of nonbiological and socioeconomic factors versus biological factors in producing them.

Racial-Ethnic Differences in Health

Race-Ethnicity as a Social Construction

Racial-ethnic differences are sizable and pervasive across time, space, and health outcomes in the United States and other countries. Race can be defined as a grouping of people who share genetically transmitted physical characteristics such as skin and hair color. But how given physical characteristics are used to categorize people, and with what consequences, is socially determined or constructed. In the United States, we historically have characterized people dichotomously as white or black, based on the "one-drop rule," a standard by which a person judged to have one ancestor who can be classified as sub-Saharan African can be considered black. This standard is currently shifting as a widening range of racial and ethnic groups immigrate to this country and as intermingling and intermarriage among them increases. The U.S. Census Bureau now allows individuals to classify themselves as being of multiple races or ethnicities. Other nations, such as Brazil and even Mexico, have recognized many variations in skin color, and in some places, such as Hawaii, race and skin color are less important bases of social differentiation.

Similarly, the social consequences of being classified as black have varied greatly depending on the time and place. In the United States, the social labels "colored," "Negro," "black," and "African American," and the meanings associated with them, have varied dramatically over time and place, though racial inequalities persist. Thus, race is for most purposes a social construct and grouping, not a biological one.

Ethnicity can be defined as a grouping of people based on culture or national origin (and occasionally religion) and is sometimes conflated or linked with race. But even more clearly than for race, ethnicity is a sociocultural concept or grouping. Thus, when we speak of and analyze racial-ethnic differences in health, we are dealing with sociocultural differences, not biological ones.[2]

Racial-Ethnic Health Disparities Are Largely Socioeconomic

Racial and ethnic categories have generally been socially constructed in the context of inequalities in resources and power, and often as a means for justifying them. Consequently, race and ethnicity are often highly correlated with, indeed determinative of, socioeconomic position. Thus, it is essential to understand the degree to which racial-ethnic disparities are mediated or explained by socioeconomic position versus other nonbiological factors.

Table 5.1 provides a simple illustration of the way socioeconomic position and race-ethnicity combine to influence health—in this case, differences in life expectancy at age forty-five by race and income (and also by gender, considered more fully shortly). Income differences are almost always larger than differences by race, especially among men, and adjustment for socioeconomic position generally reduces the racial differences (3.7 years among women and 4.9 among men) by 50 percent or

Table 5.1 U.S. Life Expectancy (in Years) at Age Forty-Five, by Family Income, Race, and Gender (1980 Dollars), 1979–1991

	Females			Males		
Yearly Family Income	White	Black	Difference	White	Black	Difference
All	36.3	32.6	3.7	31.1	26.2	4.9
Less than $10,000	35.8	32.7	3.1	27.3	25.2	2.1
Less than $10,000 to $14,999	37.4	33.5	3.9	30.3	28.1	2.2
Less than $15,000 to $24,999	37.8	36.3	1.5	32.4	31.3	1.1
$25,000 or more	38.5	36.5	2.0	33.9	32.6	1.3

Source: Adapted from House and Williams (2000, table 1). © National Academy Press. Reprinted with permission. Original data from Pamuk et al (1998, data table for figure 25).

more—and again, most clearly and consistently for men. If we adjust for multiple socioeconomic factors, racial differences are reduced even further and sometimes eliminated altogether. Thus, if race was not so consequential for socioeconomic opportunity in American society (and in other societies where race plays a large role in social life), racial differences in health would be much smaller and in some cases nonexistent.[3]

As is evident in table 5.1, however, small to moderate racial differences in health, and occasionally large ones, occur within levels of socioeconomic position, and they are usually larger at lower socioeconomic levels. Race influences more than socioeconomic position and can adversely affect health at any and all socioeconomic levels. Two factors seem especially important in understanding this independent health impact of race-ethnicity: racial discrimination and segregation.

The Role of Discrimination and Segregation

Most central is the existence and experience of *discrimination* based on race-ethnicity. Historically, discrimination has been a major determinant of the socioeconomic position of African Americans and other racial-ethnic groups, and it remains so today, though civil rights policies have gradually helped to weaken this link. However, discrimination, or the mere threat of it, is also a social phenomenon and experience that produces psychological threat and stress regardless of its impact on socioeconomic position.

A growing body of research has documented the impact of actual, threatened, and even anticipated discrimination on a wide range of social, psychological, and health outcomes. Beyond its effects on socioeconomic position, discrimination and the threat or anticipation of it can affect almost all the major risk factors for health shown in figure 4.5. A thorough review of existing research by the Institute of Medicine of the National Academies of Science found consistent evidence that African Americans and other racial minorities are less likely than whites to receive the same treatment and the most medically indicated treatment for a wide range of illnesses, even when they have the same diagnoses and the same level of health insurance and access to care.[4]

Beyond such disparities in health care, African Americans and other racial-ethnic minorities are more likely to experience serious discrimination in many realms of life. This can be relatively overt, as in employment or housing discrimination or police harassment, or more subtle, as in suggestions that these groups are less capable or deserving, as reflected, for example, in tracking or lower expectations in school. These more subtle forms of discrimination can have very tangible outcomes in terms of educational performance and attainment. The cumulative experience of discrimination of all types and levels can create a pervasive experience of threat, stress, and vigilance that adversely affects performance and health (for example, elevating blood pressure) at any and all socioeconomic levels.[5] Some of my African American male colleagues with PhDs say that they generally wear a coat and tie to lessen the chance of being stopped by police. Even so, one colleague was stopped en route to his daughter's kindergarten graduation in our university town, just because there had been a bank robbery in which the suspects were black. Unfortunately, such experiences are all too common.

One of the most important consequences of discrimination, in conjunction with governmental housing policies, is residential *segregation* of racial-ethnic groups, with concomitant educational and sometimes occupational segregation. Residential segregation usually is based on and involves discrimination and further restricts socioeconomic opportunities. But it exerts other adverse effects on health by increasing exposure to various health risk factors, such as environmental hazards, widespread advertising and sale of alcohol and tobacco, and access to illicit drugs, as well as by limiting access to health-promoting resources, from high-quality medical care to healthful food and places to walk and exercise.[6]

Both discrimination and segregation have been shown to potentially explain blacks' poor standing on health outcomes. That high blood pressure, or hypertension, persists among blacks, even in the face of successful efforts to diagnose and treat those with this condition, may be explained by the overt as well as more subtle discrimination in all aspects of life for the black population. Residential segregation especially tends to confine blacks, even those of higher socioeconomic position, to segregated neighborhoods with the kind of conditions conducive to high

Figure 5.1 A Conceptual Framework for Understanding Social Inequalities in Health and Aging by Race-Ethnicity, Gender, Age, and Socioeconomic Position

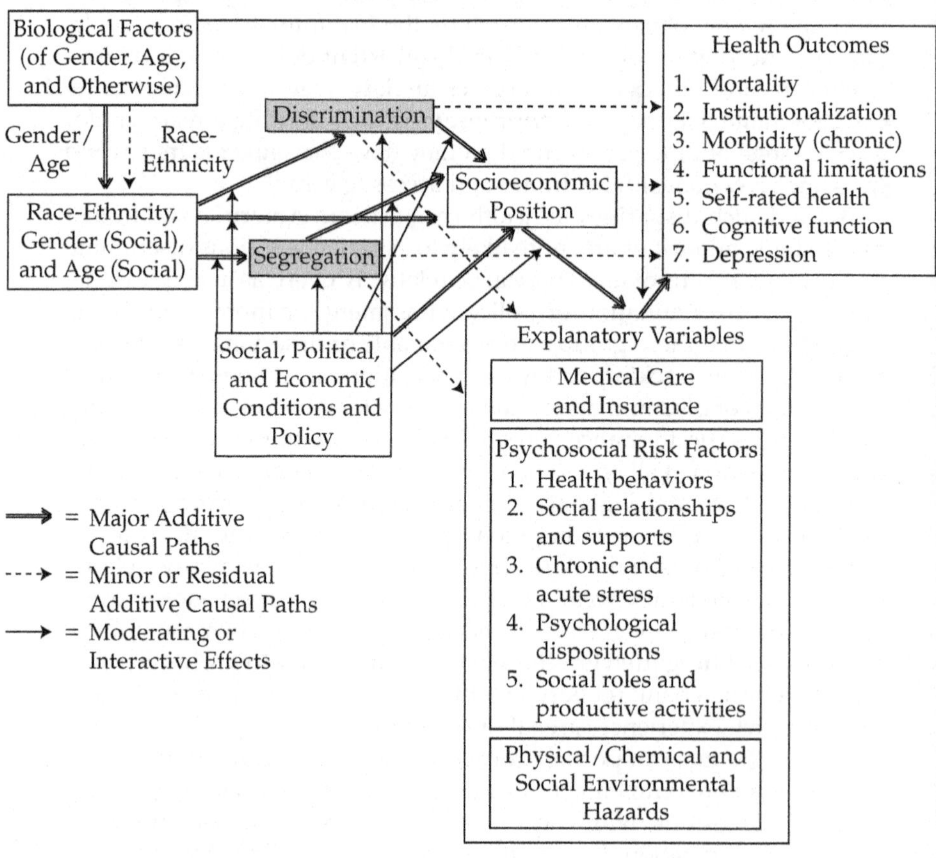

Source: Adapted from House (2002, figure 5).

blood pressure—from air pollution to the stress of physically or socially unsafe streets and homes.[7]

Figure 5.1 expands figure 4.5 (as largely indicated by shading) to indicate how and why race and ethnicity exert powerful negative effects on health not only via socioeconomic position but also via discrimination and segregation that can operate at any and all socioeconomic levels. We have the most evidence of such effects for African Americans, but researchers are increasingly documenting similar phenomena and outcomes in Latino and other populations of color.

It should be noted that minority populations of color also manifest adaptations that are beneficial and protective of their health. African

Americans, for example, are the most religious subgroup of the American population, and aspects of religion are protective of health. Most notably, those who attend religious services regularly (more than once a month) live longer than those who do not.[8] Strong community and family bonds seem to have similar health-protective effects in Latino and Asian American populations. Thus, on some indicators of health, such as depression among African Americans or physical health among Latinos, minority populations of color sometimes manifest higher levels of health than might be expected on the basis of their socioeconomic position.[9]

In sum, although existing evidence is less extensive and more complex than what we have seen for socioeconomic position, race-ethnicity constitutes another fundamental cause of social disparities in health, especially for African Americans, Native Americans, and later-generation, acculturated members of Latino and some Asian immigrant groups. Further, the bases of these disparities are primarily sociocultural rather than biological.

Gender and Health

Matters are even more complex when it comes to health differences between men and women. The distinction between them is clearly grounded in real and manifest biological differences: there is rarely ambiguity at birth in classifying a newborn's sex. However, what it means to be male or female is also heavily shaped by sociocultural forces, and sexual orientation can and sometimes does change over the life course. Thus, social and biomedical scientists increasingly speak of gender as the "socially constructed rules, behaviors, activities, and attributes that a given society considers appropriate for men and women."[10] Both the biological (anatomical and physiological) differences between sexes and the social differences between genders are critical factors in shaping the health of men and women and the disparities between them.

These complexities have resulted in the seeming paradox in most societies that women live longer than men but are more likely to suffer from many forms of illness and functional limitation. At least one reason for this paradox, historically, is that men have been more prone than women to cardiovascular disease (CVD) and lung and respiratory cancers, which are often fatal but less likely to result in prolonged illness, functional limitations, or disability prior to death. Women are protected against CVD by hormonal differences prior to menopause, and until recently they have been less exposed to the major causes of respiratory disease via conditions of work or cigarette smoking. In contrast, women suffer more often than men from non-life-threatening chronic diseases that tend to have a lengthy and more debilitating course, such as arthritis and osteoporosis.

Growing Evidence of Worsening Life Expectancy for Women

In spite of women's historically longer life expectancy, as we have seen in chapter 1, their life expectancy in the contemporary United States has been deteriorating relative both to American men and to women in comparably developed countries. Indeed, it is not implausible that American women's life expectancy could absolutely decline over the coming decades, as it already has in some places and among some portions of the population. The leveling off of gains in life expectancy for American women began about 1980, but only in the last ten to fifteen years has it become clear that this is a major long-term shift in health trajectories, not just a momentary blip produced by some more time-limited event, such as the rise and fall of hormone replacement therapy. Thus, at best, only partial explanations of these trends are possible at this time.

One compelling set of factors may lie in the changing nature of the life course of women. As women's life expectancy and advantage relative to men has increased over most of the twentieth century, women have gotten closer to the biological limits of the human life span. As the postmenopausal share of their total life expectancy has grown, the relative contribution of premenopausal protective hormonal factors to their total life expectancy has been steadily reduced. These changes in the life course have occurred for women in all societies; as illustrated in figures 1.1 to 1.5, the rate of increase in life expectancy for women relative to men has declined across the most-developed societies. The notable exception is Japan, a country where coronary heart disease, the disease most protected against by female estrogen hormones, accounts for a much smaller share of total mortality.[11]

Smoking and Health in Men Versus Women

The distinctively worsening life expectancy of American women relative both to American men and to women in other societies must be explained by other factors. The most clearly identified cause is the later growth of cigarette smoking, and hence its health impact, in women relative to men. As shown in figure 5.2, the prevalence of cigarette smoking among men reached 40 percent by 1920, peaked at 60 percent around 1960, and dropped by half (to 30 percent) by 1990. In contrast, the prevalence of smoking among women reached a peak level of about 33 percent around 1965, remained around or above 30 percent until 1980, and then declined by only about one-third (to 20 percent) by the beginning of the twenty-first century. Thus, before 1920 men reached the peak smoking rate ever achieved by women and then reduced their levels from almost twice the rate of women in 1960 to an absolute difference of about 5 percent (or about 15 percent greater than women) by 1980.

Figure 5.2 Male and Female Smoking Prevalence in the United States, 1900–2004

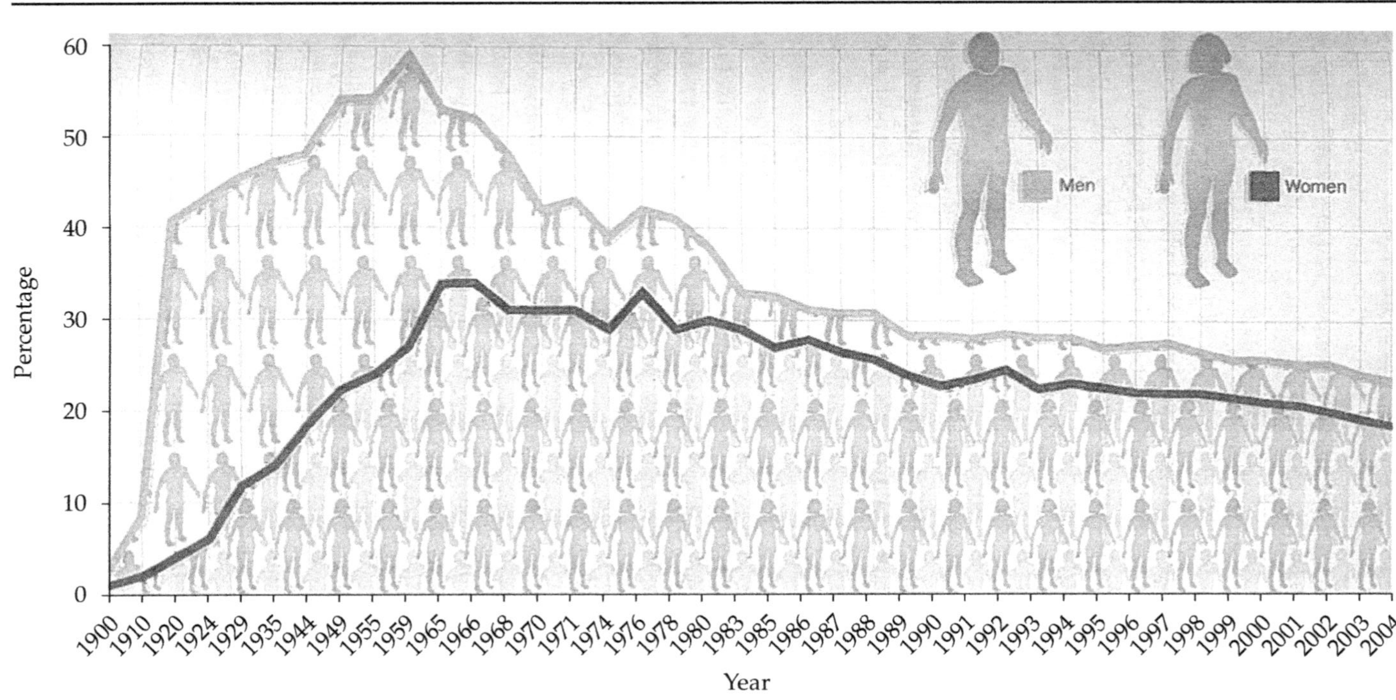

Sources: Centers for Disease Control, Surgeon General's Reports (1988, 1989, 2001), reprinted in Brandt (2007, 309).

Cigarette smoking had its greatest impact on men's health in the United States between 1955 and 1970, when increases in male life expectancy were relatively flat. In contrast, the impact of smoking has been increasingly felt among women since the 1980s and will continue to be felt strongly for another decade or more. This impact will tend to keep rates of growth in women's life expectancy at the lower level of the past few decades for at least another one or two decades, and it may even contribute to driving down the absolute levels of life expectancy for growing fractions of the female population. On the other hand, if women's smoking levels ever decline as sharply as men's did between the mid-1960s and the early 1980s, this could substantially mitigate the worsening trends in the life expectancy of American women.

The effects of smoking may have been compounded by problems in women's health care—for example, the failure to recognize or adequately respond to cardiovascular disease in women. Though less common in women than men, CVD still constitutes the greatest cause of death for women, in whom CVD may often manifest differently and at different ages than for men.

Declining Women's Health: Social but Not Only Socioeconomic

There have almost certainly been other factors adversely affecting American women's health over the past few decades and helping to account for why women are doing so poorly relative not only to American men but also to women in other societies. These factors are likely to continue to operate for decades to come. Whereas socioeconomic factors clearly account for many of the racial-ethnic disparities in health—and sometimes all of them—because their relation to gender is complex, they only partially explain gender disparities in health.

Traditionally, most American women were not in the paid labor force. Their socioeconomic position (SEP) mainly derived from the SEP of their husband or family; the latter continues to be positively associated with women's health. As women have entered the paid labor force in greater numbers, however, their own education, occupation, income, and wealth have come to be equally and increasingly more predictive of their health than the SEP of their spouse or family. Historically, women have lagged behind men in their socioeconomic attainments, but these gaps are closing. Younger age cohorts of women now exceed men in educational attainment and are likely to continue to close the occupational, income, and wealth gaps. Thus, on average, as socioeconomic position affects women and men in increasingly similar ways, it appears to be less and less consequential for understanding gender disparities in health. At the same time, the growth of single-parent families, almost entirely headed by women, is creating a subgroup of women who are disadvantaged socioeconomically, and perhaps also in levels of smoking, relative to both men and other women. Further, they may experience more intensively other stresses that affect all women, ranging from actual and perceived discrimination to managing a high level of stress in combining occupational, parental, and household responsibilities, particularly around caregiving for both younger and older generations. The role of all these changes and stresses in the overall declining health of women has yet to be adequately studied and understood.[12]

The gender revolution that has greatly equalized women's educational and occupational lives relative to men has not been accompanied by commensurate alteration of the distribution of responsibilities and work in marriage, family life, and child-rearing. Such alterations could be made either by redistributing the domestic work responsibilities of men and women or by redistributing resources and supports from the private to the public sector, as has occurred much more in other developed societies—for example, through universal access to postmaternity leave, child care, and early childhood education. It has been hypothesized, but not clearly and definitively shown, that the "second job" of most women—more and more of them without a spouse or partner to share the load—adversely affects their health. And just as the effects of cigarette smoking took twenty to thirty years to build up and hence clearly manifest themselves, the same may be true of the great changes in gender roles at the end of the twentieth century. They may already be manifesting in the increasing mortality rates of older cohorts of women who: (1) have had labor force experiences that were less positive than those of younger cohorts; (2) have found themselves working two jobs in the "sandwich" stage of the life course as they care for both children and aging parents with little or no help from spouses or partners; and (3) are caring for the children and parents of a second spouse or partner, with whom women are more likely now than in the past to be living. We may also be able to learn from more intensive study of populations of women who have experienced this constellation of conditions of life and work over most of their history, such as African American women.

Gender as an Increasingly Social Determinant of Health

Just as we have come to understand that differences in the social roles and behavior of men and women are much more socially constructed than driven by biology, we have also recognized that health differences between men and women are socially determined as well. The lingering impact of the later rise and then slower decline in smoking among women is one such difference. (Other health behaviors, such as overweight and obesity, may come to have similar effects.) In all realms of life, women, like racial-ethnic groups, face discrimination—and even segregation in some realms, especially occupations—that can adversely affect their health. In addition, via the pathways illustrated in figure 5.1, the distribution of rights and responsibilities within and across the vocational and domestic spheres of life may be negatively affecting women's health. At the same time, women continue to have an advantage over men in certain health-protective factors, from their hormonal makeup to their generally less physically and clinically hazardous occupational exposures to the better quantity or quality of their social relationships.

Aging as Both a Social and Biological Process

It is not often that we consider age in the context of social disparities in health. Yet age is in many ways comparable and related to race-ethnicity, gender, and socioeconomic position as a dimension of such disparities. Like sex, age is an intrinsically biological phenomenon. As we saw in figure 4.4, health and functioning vary by age in highly biological as well as socially determined ways.

But even age has become substantially socially constructed and determined. The periods of the life course we now label as "adolescence" and "young adulthood" were not viewed as such until the last couple of centuries. Persons of those ages, as well as some we would now consider "children," were in many ways and places treated as (often shorter) adults, including the expectation that they would do both paid and unpaid labor that is now limited to adults. This remains the social construction of childhood and adolescence in some developing countries. Similarly, what some now call the "third age"—an increasingly extended period of life and leisure in older age without paid employment—is essentially a creation of the modern era, the result of the private and public pensions developed over the last 100 to 150 years.

Moreover, the social status, resources, power, and rights and responsibilities of children, adolescents, adults, and the elderly have been, and continue to be, highly variable across time and societies. As social and living conditions for children have improved, so has their health, life expectancy, stature, and health as adults, and these improvements in the lives and health of children have contributed to the dramatic improvements in the health of human populations over time. Similarly, as societies in the modern era recognized their responsibility to ensure reasonable conditions of life and health for the elderly, the quality of their health greatly improved, thus contributing significantly to the continuing improvements in life expectancy and population health in developed societies. In sum, age is another axis of social stratification and inequality within and across societies that needs to be considered in conjunction with ethnicity, gender, and socioeconomic position.

Socioeconomic Position and Age

As with race-ethnicity, variations in health by age that are social in nature can be substantially explained by socioeconomic factors. Most notably, the improvements in the health of the elderly have been driven, as we saw in chapter 4, not only by the increasing availability and quality of medical care but also by improvements in their socioeconomic position, especially their income as a result of Social Security and, for many, job-related pensions. Their improved economic status and resources have driven improvements in their health, both directly, via better conditions of life and work, and indirectly as they have been enabled to retire, fully or partially, from work that may have been deleterious to their health. In the United States and other developed countries, the establishment of public and private pension systems and the indexing of public ones to inflation have virtually eliminated poverty among the elderly, at least up until the Great Recession, which presented a set of issues we return to in chapter 7. These economic resources also facilitated access to and utilization of medical care. In analogous ways, the universality of health insurance for the elderly in developed countries affects their health not only directly via the medical care they receive but also indirectly by protecting them against the potential negative effects on their health of being economically depleted, or even bankrupted, by health care expenses.

Social Determinants and Disparities and the Biology of Age

Age as a biological phenomenon also conditions and contextualizes the impact of social determinants and disparities in health. Our robustness or frailty varies over the life course, constraining the impact on our health of social disparities. Disparities by socioeconomic position and by race-ethnicity and gender tend to be smallest during the periods of the life course when we are at either our most biologically robust (late adolescence and early adulthood) or our most frail (later old age). These disparities tend to be sizable in early life, become smaller through early adulthood, increase again during middle and early old age, and then diminish toward the end of life. However, as we saw in chapter 4, disparities wax and wane at constantly evolving points owing to both socio-environmental contexts and changes in medical care.

Similarly, the impact of social factors on health outcomes waxes and wanes as a function of biological changes over the life course. Women are hormonally protected against cardiovascular disease during their childbearing and -rearing years. Humans also tend to gain weight through middle and early old age, after which weight tends to decline. Thus, the factors producing the obesity epidemic—whether social or socioenvironmental—have been increasingly manifested as one moves downward in age, and now extend into adolescence—and even childhood for some populations.

In sum, one cannot think about social disparities in health without thinking about age in conjunction with the traditional socioeconomic, racial-ethnic, or gender axes of such disparities. And we need to think about all of these dimensions of social inequality together in what sociologists term an "intersectional" way.

Being Poor, Black, Female, and Young Can Be Bad for Your Health

Growing evidence indicates that occupying disadvantaged socioeconomic, racial-ethnic, and gender roles in American society can be bad—often very bad—for your health. And these effects are cumulative and even synergistic for people who are disadvantaged on all or most of these axes of inequality. Black women of lower socioeconomic status manifest at relatively early ages a burden of morbidity that far exceeds that of almost any other portion of the population. This synergistic cumulation of socioeconomic, racial-ethnic, and gender disadvantages can lead to functional problems, disability, and even relatively early death. Counterintuitively, teenage childbearing is an arguably rational response to these cumulative adverse or "weathering" effects on health. Early childbearing increases the chance that the mother and her female relatives, who often assist each other in child-rearing in disadvantaged populations, will be as healthy as possible, enhancing, in turn, the health and life chances of the child carried and then reared by the woman and her relatives.[13] Note in this effect the interaction of age with race, gender, and socioeconomic position.

This same population is now being further affected by the obesity epidemic. Increases in obesity have been surprisingly similar across socioeconomic, racial-ethnic, and gender lines for most of the population. However, in young adult (and probably also adolescent) portions of the population—those at the ages when weight gain tends, for biological reasons, to be greatest—a striking social disparity in weight gain has become evident. No segment of the American population has been able to avoid gaining weight over the past thirty years, but the lowest trajectories of weight gain in early adulthood (and probably also adolescence) have been among higher-SEP white males, as can be seen on college campuses and in the periodicals on health and fitness directed at this segment of the population. These advantaged men have even gained less on

Figure 5.3 BMI Trajectories from 1986 to 2001 of Low-Income Black Women and High-Income White Men Age Twenty-Five to Thirty-Nine in 1986

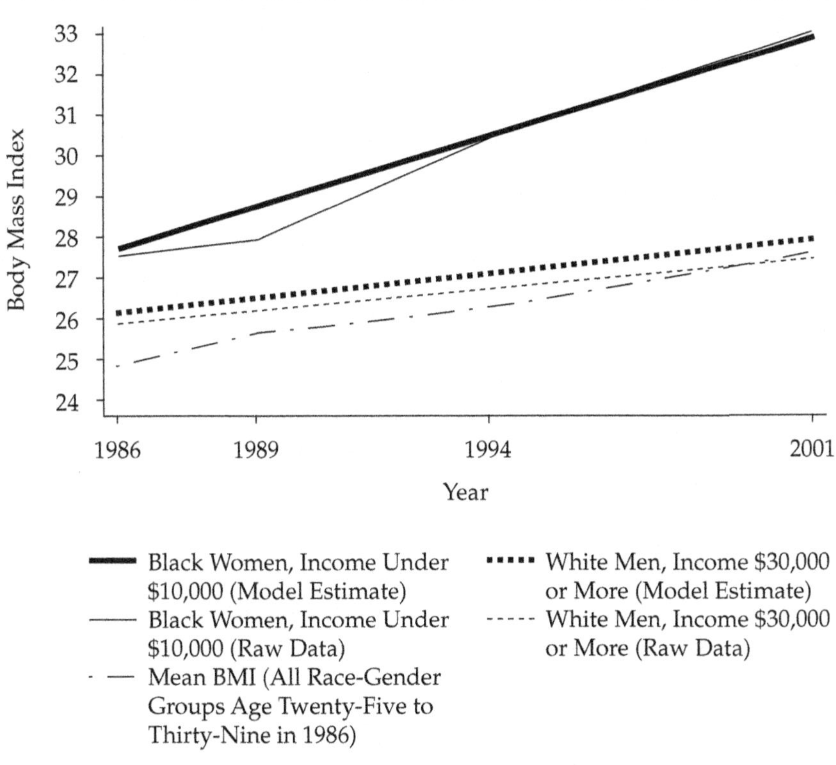

Source: Ailshire and House (2011, figure 2).
Note: All numbers are weighted.

average than high-SEP white women, who are traditionally the thinnest group in the U.S. population. In contrast, young adult, lower-SEP, black women have manifested the greatest weight gain over the past three decades: their almost five-point increase, on average, in body mass index (BMI)—the scale used to classify the body size of the population—is large enough to move an individual from the "normal" range (BMI of 25 or less) to the "obese" range (BMI of 30 or more).

These differences can be graphically seen in figure 5.3, which shows, for the nationally representative Americans' Changing Lives sample of the American population, the average BMI trajectories of low-income black women and high-income white men age twenty-five to thirty-nine in 1986 as they aged to become forty to fifty-four in 2001–2002. The BMI of the total population in this age range increased from 25 (normal weight) to about 27 (moderately overweight) between 1986 and 2001–2002. The BMI of high-income white men increased at a slightly lower rate, though it started at a higher level owing to the contribution of higher-SEP white women to holding down the overall population average in 1986. But the BMI of poor black women increased by over five points over the same period, from a little under 28 (moderately overweight) to over 33 (moderately obese). Put another way, the disparity in weight between these groups increased by 250 percent in just fifteen years.[14]

From the New Science of Health to a New Health Policy

In sum, although socioeconomic disparities are arguably the largest and most central element of social disparities in American society, both science and policy must attend to disparities by race-ethnicity, gender, and age and to the powerful and often complex ways in which these dimensions of disparities combine to affect health. Reducing the nonbiological and social bases of all of these disparities, and combinations thereof, is the single greatest action we can take to improve population health. It is also probably the single greatest action we have taken over the last several centuries to increase human health and life expectancy twice (from 1780 to 1900 and then again from 1900 to the present) by more than had been accomplished in all prior human history.[15]

We are now ready to consider the implications of the science of social determinants and disparities in health for social and health policy—and in particular for a new demand-side approach. Our discussion of social and health policy will be founded on the understandings from chapters 2 to 5 that (1) the primary determinants of health are not health care and insurance, but rather social, environmental, psychological, and behavioral factors; (2) the main way we can improve population health—and increasingly the only way—is to reduce social disparities in health by race-ethnicity, gender, even age, and especially socioeconomic position; and (3) population health will be improved not primarily by biomedical science and practice or health care reform, important as these remain, but rather by recognizing and using all social or public policy as the fundamental basis of health policy.

Part II

Policy Implications

Chapter 6

A New Demand-Side Health Policy: Implications for Research, Education, Policy, and Practice

WHAT WOULD a demand-side health policy, grounded in the science of social determinants and disparities in health, look like? And how different would it be from current supply-side approaches? Any answer to the first question must necessarily be both comprehensive and complex. The answer to the second question is "very," though a demand-side policy would strongly complement supply-side approaches, not supplant them.

Our current supply-side health policy developed via the initially sequential, now multiple and simultaneous, operation of three foundational elements: research, education, and policy and practice. A new demand-side approach will require the same foundational elements and a similar developmental process, albeit one that operates more rapidly than the processes for both supply-side health policy over the past 150 years and the demand-side approaches taken to date. The need for alternatives to current policy is immediate and will only become more pressing with each passing year.

Prior Demand-Side Approaches to Health

A demand-side approach to improving health and controlling health care expenditures is not really new. In fact, it has arguably been the major way in which population health has already been improved, and much more cost-effectively than happens with our current supply-side approach. In some of the following cases, the demand-side factors used to improve health and control or reduce the need for care were biomedical, but even more of them were non-biomedical.

The Decline of Infectious Disease

Although broader social and economic developments and related improvements in public health probably played a considerably larger role in the decline of infectious disease (as we saw in chapter 3), the development and application of pharmacological vaccination and treatment, a demand-side approach, effectively established the hegemony of modern biomedical science and practice. The thrust of this biomedical approach was preventing the onset of disease in individuals, and hence populations, or failing that, providing immediate and rapid treatment to curtail or cure illness in its very early stages.

Between 1900 and 1950 in the United States, the combined effect of social and economic development, public health measures, and biomedical practice was to increase life expectancy by almost twenty-two years, while raising the proportion of gross domestic product spent on health from probably less than 1 percent to about 4 percent. In contrast, as discussed in chapters 2 and 3, the quadrupling of expenditures on health care since that era has had a rapidly diminishing rate of return—producing a further gain in life expectancy of only about ten years. There are, of course, gains in quality of life that stem from improvements in health care's ability to manage the progression of diseases and alleviate some of their adverse effects, such as pain and impaired functioning.

Dental Public Health

Dentistry provides the most dramatic single example of a demand-side approach to improving population health while controlling or even reducing health care expenditures. From its early days, the dental profession has placed considerable emphasis on trying to prevent the onset of dental disease. This was perhaps because, in contrast to medical treatment, which often relieved immediate and short-term patient pain and suffering, dental treatment, such as filling cavities, often occurred in early or asymptomatic stages of disease, creating pain and suffering in the interest of longer-term dental health (maintenance and retention of healthy teeth and gums). Thus, dentistry has always stressed regular prophylaxis, cleaning, and examination of teeth and surrounding tissue and supported efforts to promote dental health via general public health approaches.

Dentistry was also able to identify a kind of silver public health bullet: the application of low-level fluoride to developing teeth in childhood, most cost-effectively by adding fluoride to public drinking water and to toothpaste. In spite of substantial initial public opposition during the 1940s and 1950s, the dental profession eventually succeeded in achieving widespread exposure to low levels of fluoride, with consequent substantial reduction and even elimination of dental caries (cavities). Whereas my grandfather had only dentures during the last decades of his life and my parents had heavily filled, crowned, and bridged teeth, my brother and I have had a relatively low level of cavities and subsequent dental problems, and our children have virtually none. These personal experiences are confirmed by population data, which show that the average number of decayed, missing, and filled permanent teeth in children age six to eighteen in the United States has declined by 57.2 percent, from 4.44 in the early 1970s to 1.90 in the early 1990s, with 50 percent of children free of dental caries by the 1990s.[1]

We do not have good data on total expenditures for dental care in the United States, although the growth of the dental profession provides one crude indicator. Since the early 1990s, the number of dentists (per 100,000 population) has declined slightly and is projected to continue to do so through 2026.[2] The orientation of dental insurance has also changed: it now is likely to focus on and most completely cover preventive services. Serious social disparities in dental health and access to dental care continue to exist. Nevertheless, dentistry provides a worthy example of how demand-side-focused health policy can both improve health and control or reduce expenditures for care, especially nondiscretionary care.

Recent Improvements in Population Health

While the population health of the United States has declined relative to other countries, it has continued to improve absolutely. And the areas of greatest progress further illustrate the importance of demand-side approaches, most commonly via "nonhealth" policy. As always, this progress also reflects complementary improvements in medical care.

Figure 6.1 shows death rates from the five current leading causes of death over the past half-century. The biggest declines have come in cardiovascular disease and cerebrovascular disease (largely stroke). Efforts to determine the cause of these trends, though difficult, consistently suggest that in the United States and Europe probably less than half of these declines can be attributed to medical care. The majority are a product of the declines in risk factors, such as smoking, high cholesterol, and high blood pressure, that accompany changes in lifestyle. Most important have been declines in cigarette smoking, improvements in dietary patterns (consumption of less saturated fat and more fiber, fruits, and vegetables), and increased physical activity. Improved pharmacological treatment of blood pressure has also been important, with effective pharmacologic treatment of high cholesterol (especially via statins) a relatively late development.[3]

Changes in smoking, diet, and exercise have been driven by broader population-based strategies for changing behaviors, such as taxation on

Figure 6.1 Age-Adjusted Death Rates by Major Causes, 1960–2009

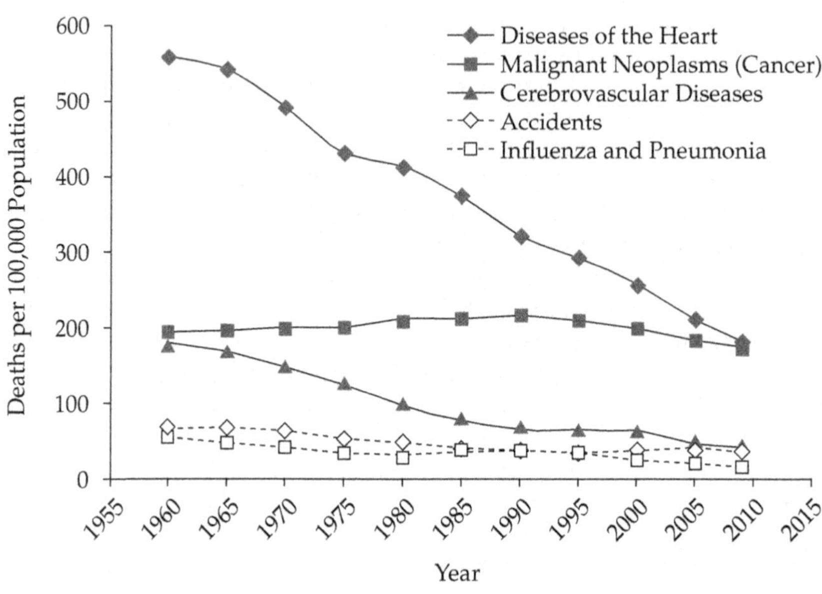

Sources: Author compilation based on U.S. Census Bureau (2012) and Kochanek et al. (2011, table B).

cigarettes and restrictions on advertising and places where people can smoke, increased availability of low-fat products and dietary guidelines (for high cholesterol), and promotion of physical activity by both the public and private sectors.

The modest decline in accidental deaths has been a function mainly of large declines in motor vehicle deaths, which have occurred even as the amount of driving has increased. Mainly owing to improvements in highway and motor vehicle design, laws mandating the use of seat belts and child safety restraints, and efforts to reduce drunk driving and improve driver training and regulation, especially of younger drivers, the decline in motor vehicle deaths per million miles driven has been very dramatic, from 5.5 in 1966 to 1.1 in 2010.[4] The declines in influenza and pneumonia have been primarily attributable to improved vaccines and access to them, reminiscent of earlier declines in some infectious diseases.

In contrast to the other major causes of death, mortality rates for cancer, which has had the largest National Institutes of Health (NIH) research budget and a proliferation of new treatments, have declined only slightly and recently, and those declines largely reflect earlier detection. The greatest declines have been in respiratory cancer, a result of the decline in cigarette smoking (see figures 3.1 and 5.2).

The Power of Demand-Side Approaches

Historically, then, we have already seen the power of demand-side policies—utilizing largely nonmedical practices to prevent or postpone the onset of infections and dental and chronic diseases—both to improve population health and to mitigate the utilization of and expenditures for health care. In a world in which social disparities in health constitute not only the biggest drags on population health but also the greatest opportunities for improving it, policies that reduce socioeconomic deprivations and their behavioral and psychological sequelae could plausibly be the foundation of a new demand-side policy for improving health, largely through nonhealth factors and policies. At the same time, such policies could control or reduce expenditures for health care and insurance. Chapters 7 and 9 discuss the most promising policies, and chapter 8 shows that they can significantly reduce health care expenditures.

The foundation for all of these demand-side approaches has been twofold: (1) basic research that identified the biomedical and non-biomedical factors that could powerfully reduce the incidence and prevalence of diseases or accidents; and (2) the development of educational programs for training health care and other professionals in translating these basic research findings into practice and policy to prevent the onset of illness and injury and hence cost-effectively promote health and constrain expenditures for health care and insurance. We now need just as profound a transformation of health research, education, practice, and policy as occurred in the late nineteenth and early twentieth centuries. However, this transformation must be based as much or more on the social, psychological, behavioral, and environmental sciences as on biomedical sciences.

Research

As we saw in chapter 3, modern biomedical science, education, and practice and policy evolved in the late nineteenth and early twentieth centuries from major advances in bacteriologic and virologic science. Those scientific developments led to a codification of modern biomedical science and education that, for better or for worse, essentially swept aside all competitors, including the incipient social medicine of the mid-nineteenth century.

Rebalancing Biomedical Research and Research in Social Determinants and Disparities

As we also saw in chapters 3 to 5, a science of social determinants and disparities in health has been developing since the mid-twentieth century, and this science is the foundation for new demand-side approaches to health research, education, practice, and policy. Currently, however, research on social determinants and disparities in health remains dwarfed by biomedical research—as can be seen in the patterns of research funding by the National Institutes of Health, the nation's major center and source of research on health. Figure 6.2 shows that the growth rate of the NIH budget since 1950 has exceeded even the growth rate of overall spending on health. The NIH budget has more or less doubled over each decade since 1950, an annual compounded growth of about 7 percent per year (in actual dollars, not adjusted for inflation) if the growth were even across the years. In fact, a major chunk of this growth occurred when Congress doubled the NIH budget between 1998 and 2003; post-2003 increments have been largely at or below the rate of inflation. Currently, NIH faces much the same fiscal limitations and uncertainties as all other federal agencies and departments, especially in its discretionary spending as opposed to the entitlement components of its budget.

Only since 1996, when the Office of Behavioral and Social Sciences Research was created within the NIH Director's Office, has there been a consistent effort to identify the portion of NIH funding that goes for behavioral and social sciences research (BSSR). Since 1996, funding for all BSSR has constituted, more or less constantly, about 10 percent of the total NIH budget, and it probably was at this level or lower in prior years.

Notable in figure 6.2 is a growing absolute gap in spending for biomedical research relative to BSSR: from a difference of about $11 billion in 1996–1997 to a difference of between $25.5 billion and $27.5 billion between 2006 and 2009, during which period BSSR funding essentially did not increase. Thus, during times of sometimes quite large increases in the NIH budget, no effort was made to increase the proportional share of funds for the new area of BSSR. Further, in the recent period of stagnation in NIH funding, BSSR funding has not even increased proportionally with the NIH budget—indeed, it has not increased at all—and has thus declined in real (inflation-adjusted) value.[5] Finally, NIH has *declined* to support critical research for a demand-side health policy grounded in understanding the social determinants of and disparities in health—specifically, the final recommendation of the National Research Council and Institute of Medicine panel report, *Shorter Lives, Poorer Health,* that NIH support research on the health impacts of nonhealth policies.[6]

The imbalance between BSSR and biomedical research support is even larger in the private sector. The research and development programs of pharmaceutical, medical equipment and supplies, and biotechnology companies constitute a growth sector that is almost entirely biomedically focused, with a small effort put into programs for supporting "wellness"

Figure 6.2 National Institutes of Health Budget, 1950–2010: Total Budget and Behavioral and Social Sciences Research Budget

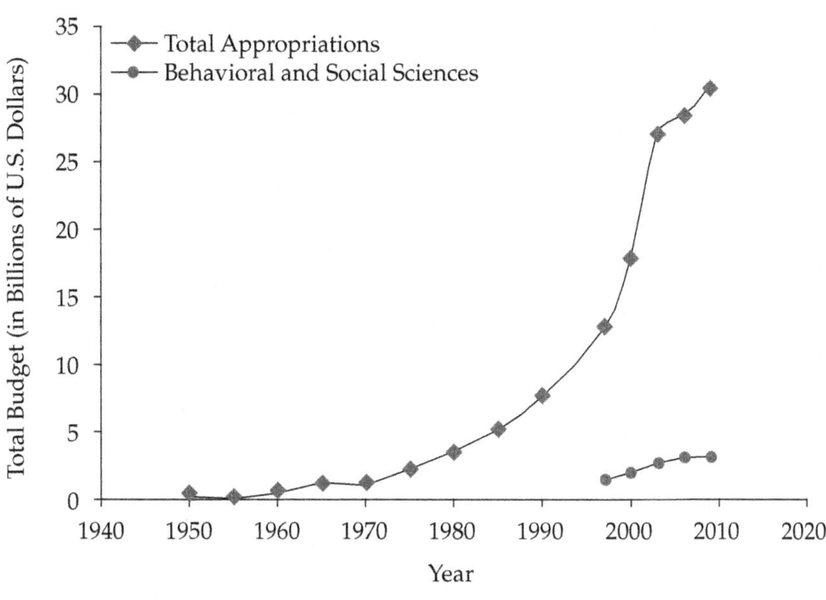

Sources: NIH, Office of Budget (various years) and NIH, Office of Behavioral and Social Sciences Research (2005, 2008).

or health-promoting behavior. Similarly, health-related private philanthropy, whether from individuals or foundations, is also heavily focused on biomedical research, though some research in the areas of social determinants and disparities in health has been developed, particularly at the Robert Wood Johnson Foundation.

Thus, one major component of a new demand-side approach to health policy must be a rebalancing of health research, moving it from its perpetual biomedical focus toward a greatly enhanced focus on social and behavioral determinants of health. Given the growing budgetary pressure on research spending in both the public and private sectors, funds from biomedical agendas may have to be reallocated to other agendas. Just as health care reform is promoting more cost-benefit analysis of medical care via comparative effectiveness research, a similar lens needs to be focused on the relative costs and benefits of all aspects of health research. Such a focus could lead to a reallocation of funds from biomedical research with low returns in terms of health outcomes toward health research—social, environmental, psychological, and behavioral as well as biomedical—with higher returns. This would include more funding for the kind of research reviewed in chapters 3 to 5 and for the basic social science underpinnings of such research, as well as for the new forms of policy-oriented psychosocial research discussed in this and the next two chapters.

Rebalancing Disease-Focused Research and Cause-Focused Research

Modern biomedical research on chronic diseases is still largely driven by the disease-specific model that was developed in the age of infectious disease in the hope of finding specific causes and hence solutions for specific diseases. Thus, from its inception just before and after World War II, NIH has been largely organized into a set of disease (cluster)-specific institutes: cancer (1937); heart, lung, and blood diseases (1948); skeletal and craniofacial disorders (1948); allergy and infectious diseases (1948); diabetes, digestive, and kidney diseases (1948); mental health (1948); and neurological disorders and stroke (1950). In 1962 NIH assumed major responsibility for funding basic biological science via the National Institute of General Medical Sciences, which initially constituted 10 to 15 percent of NIH's budget. In time this proportion declined by about half (to 6 to 7 percent), though the institute has been supplemented since the late 1980s and early 1990s by the 1 to 2 percent of the NIH budget devoted to the Human Genome Institute. Together these nine basic biological and specific disease-oriented institutes continue to account for over two-thirds of NIH's total budget.

The rest of the NIH budget is distributed among the other institutes founded since 1962: five disease-focused institutes (alcohol and alcoholism, arthritis and musculoskeletal and skin, deafness and communications disorders, drug abuse, and eye), two focused on stages of the life course (childhood and aging), two focused on specific health professions (nursing and biomedical engineering), and two focused (like the genome project) on the general causes of many diseases (environment and minority status).Thus, over 70 percent of NIH's budget is concentrated in the twelve disease-specific research institutes, and only 11 percent goes to the four institutes (general medical science, human genome, environmental health, and minority health and health disparities) that focus on general causes and processes of health and disease. The two life-course institutes combine disease-specific approaches with general cause or process approaches.

Interestingly, only about one-third of the variance in NIH funding across specific diseases can be predicted by the actual mortality, morbidity, and disability burden of these diseases in the population. Thus, even in the biomedical arena, NIH research funding appears to be only crudely targeted.[7]

NIH research should quite arguably be organized as much around *causes* of disease as disease outcomes. The determinants of chronic diseases tend not to be disease-specific, but rather affect a wide range of disease outcomes. This is certainly true of social, environmental, and behavioral causes of disease. Although some environmental factors, such as exposure to specific chemicals, may have relatively disease-specific effects, most do not. Pollution affects respiratory, cardiovascular, and cancer disease outcomes. Smoking has similarly broad effects, as do exercise, nutrition and obesity, and alcohol consumption. And as seen in figures 4.6 to 4.8, socioeconomic position, race-ethnicity, and gender affect a wide range of health outcomes and risk factors. Thus, NIH should complement its disease-specific organization and focus with a focus on major causes, devoting greater attention to social and behavioral causes of disease in particular. One can imagine institutes being refocused on health behaviors; socioeconomic factors (perhaps combined with racial-ethnic and other sources of social disparities and inequalities); social relationships and supports; and psychological factors—or focused on some combination of these areas, as in the Swedish National Institute for Psychosocial Factors in Health. Somewhat like the existing genome and general medicine science institutes, each of these reconstituted institutes could focus on a wide range of disease outcomes. Similarly, NIH needs to support basic social, psychological, and behavioral research as much as basic biological research; and programs need to be targeted on the interaction between social-environmental-behavioral and biological factors, such as gene-environment interactions.[8]

In sum, a fundamental requisite for reshaping health policy to be more demand-focused is refocusing research toward broader determinants of health—social, environmental, psychological, and behavioral as well as biomedical. And it is especially important that we reshape policy to focus not only on how such factors generate disease but also on how they promote health and prevent disease.

Education

As discussed in chapter 3, the Flexner Report institutionalized in the early twentieth century an already developing model of education for physicians and other health professionals grounded almost exclusively in basic biological and physiological sciences and their applications to specific clinical diseases. Thus, these basic sciences (and their necessary underpinnings in chemistry and physics) became the focus of both premedical postsecondary education and the initial period of professional study in schools of medicine and other health professions. The later years are devoted to clinical training, organized (with the exception of primary care fields) largely by organ- or disease-specific medical specialties.

Some things have changed in the century since the release of the Flexner Report, but not nearly to the degree that they should if we are to have a serious demand-side approach to health policy. The prerequisites for admission to medical school are courses in biology, physics, and chemistry (introductory and organic), along with English. The prerequisites added by specific schools are also generally in the natural or life sciences and math (for example, biochemistry, genetics, calculus, or statistics). The Medical College Admission Test focuses on the same areas. Although medical schools increasingly suggest that students explore and major in other areas as undergraduates, the majority still major in biology or related areas of science or math.

Once in medical school, the basic science curriculum is almost entirely biomedical, including basic courses such as anatomy, physiology, histology, biochemistry, embryology, and neuroscience in the first year and courses in medically applied areas, such as pathology, pharmacology, microbiology, and immunology, the second year. At various times and places, medical schools have added courses in human behavior, most of them related to issues of mental health and the processes and organization of medical care and patient-provider interaction. Little or no course work is required, however, on the broader socioenvironmental and psychological and behavioral contexts and causations of health and disease and of disease prevention, either prior to or in medical school. And clinical education, like research, is organized largely by organ and disease specialties.[9]

Much the same is true in allied health professions such as pharmacology and nursing, although nursing and medical social work are becoming more likely to consider the broader contexts from which patients come and in which they live and work. Even public health has taken an increasingly biomedical and disease-specific form and focus in the early twenty-first century, and consideration of broader socioenvironmental determinants of health is still variable across schools of public health and their subareas and departments.

Thus, the vast bulk of health professionals have had little exposure to, much less in-depth understanding of, the kinds of health determinants considered in chapters 3 to 5. This gap in their education limits even their purely clinical roles, but as indicated in chapter 3, clinical practitioners are becoming more aware from their own experience that important determinants of health, and hence ways of promoting and maintaining health, lie beyond their biomedical training and skills.

Because health professionals generally occupy the key administrative positions with respect to health policy at all levels of the public and private sectors and often play significant roles in legislative bodies, especially in relation to health policy, the limitations in their training are even more consequential. Frequently lacking a broad liberal arts training or training in the social epidemiology of health and illness, few health profession leaders are predisposed to consider, formulate, and implement a broader and arguably more cost-effective demand-side approach to health policy. We badly need a twenty-first century version of the Flexner Report that would reform the education of health professionals in light of the last half-century's research on social determinants and disparities in health, just as Flexner did in 1910 in bringing to light the then still seminal developments of bacteriologic and virologic science of the late nineteenth and early twentieth centuries.

What we do *not* need is any immediate effort to reduce the influence of biomedically trained health professionals in health policy. Unfortunately most social scientists are currently no more capable of understanding and utilizing the science of chapters 3 to 5 in formulating health policy, and perhaps are less so. For example, most economists, the most prominent social scientists in public policy education and practice, see biomedical science and practice as the technological basis of the production of health, comparable to the technologies that underlie and advance the production of other desired economic outcomes. Thus, health economics is largely about improving the operation of the health care and insurance system; economists pay only minor (if increasing) attention to social determinants and disparities in health. Much the same is true of health psychology and behavioral medicine, and even a good number of those in health and medical sociology take a view similar to that of the economists. The fundamental importance of social determinants and disparities in health for resolving America's paradoxical crisis of health care and health needs to be understood by a broader range of both social and biomedical scientists.

Health Practice and Policy

Just as health research and education need to be greatly reoriented, so must health policy and practice. And just as research has taught us that health care and insurance are not the main determinants of health, so we must also recognize that health policy cannot and should not be mainly health care and insurance policy. Rather, the predominant sources of population health, and its changes and disparities, are all the other "nonhealth" aspects of policy in the public and private sectors. Indeed, some broad areas of nonhealth policy, such as socioeconomic policy, may be even more important determinants of health than the current health policy.

This idea has begun to be recognized in discussion and theorizing about public policy, though in very limited, imperfect, and not yet consequential ways to date. The critical role of nonhealth policy has especially been embodied in two new concepts: health impact assessment (HIA) and health in all policies (HiAP).

Health Impact Assessment

The idea behind health impact assessment is that all policies have potential health impacts that need to be assessed and taken into account in all areas of public and private policy. The idea and its label are analogous to the concept of the environmental impact assessment (EIA), which rose out of the growing recognition over the last half of the twentieth century that all aspects of public and private behavior and policy may affect the environment physically, chemically, biologically, or socially, and often quite severely. Thus, it became critical when considering any public or private priority or policy to also assess its environmental impacts. Only then could the full costs and benefits of a policy or practice be factored into the implicit or explicit cost-benefit analysis driving policy decisions.

As a result of this insight, even things that were clearly beneficial to health in some ways came to be questioned. For instance, widespread application of DDT to control infection-carrying mosquitoes and other insects, and hence reduce the spread of serious and often fatal diseases such as malaria and West Nile influenza, had such adverse effects on the health of humans and especially on other species and the broader ecological environment that the program was ultimately halted and the pesticide banned. Today an EIA is required for many non-environmental policies before they can be put in place, and as a result some of them are modified or even eliminated. However, the assessments sometimes provide evidence of the benefits of existing policies originally enacted for other reasons. For example, the development of renewable energy not only increases overall energy supplies and reduces the demand, cost, and use of carbon-based energy but may also improve air quality and reduce global warming. If the latter benefits are sufficiently large, the health effects of renewable energy may make it more cost-effective than conventional carbon-based energy sources, even if renewable energy sources cost more than carbon-energy production.

From EIA to HIA

Environmental impact assessment remains controversial, but the practice is also widespread and consequential in policymaking in many non-environmental arenas. In contrast, health impact assessment is in its infancy and has yet to have any major impact on public policy with respect to health or other areas. Chapter 7 will focus on evidence for the health benefits and costs of a range of public policies that should alter our approach not only to health policy but also to policy in nonhealth areas. Taking into account the health impact of nonhealth policies could radically alter our cost-benefit analyses of many current public policy proposals and discussions, from Medicare, private health insurance, Social Security, and private pensions to other areas of discretionary public and private spending.[10]

Health in All Policies

Some policymakers in both the public and private sectors—more so in Europe than in the United States—have come to recognize that social determinants of health are probably more important than biomedical determinants, and that social disparities in health represent not only a social injustice but also a notable impediment to further improvements in overall population health. This recognition has been reflected in the growing number of proposals to improve population health and reduce social disparities in health that come under the rubric of "health in all policies."

In its most comprehensive and ambitious formulations, HiAP argues that since health is more often determined by factors and policies other than conventional biomedical factors and policies, the health impact of all policies should be recognized, assessed, and used in a coordinated way across policy sectors to improve population health and reduce social disparities in health. The idea is not without precedent: in many ways it informed the social medicine of Virchow over 150 years ago, and it was articulated by policymakers outside the field of health policy almost four decades ago, in 1972, when Finland's Economic Council stated:

> The measures that are used for achieving the objectives (on different levels) of health policy can not be limited only to measures within health care, but for each objective the best possible measures for reaching the objective need to be found, no matter in which sector of the public policy they belong. . . . A great number of the measures of a comprehensive (preventive) health policy are in fact the responsibility of and implemented by other public policy sectors: economic policy, employment policy, housing policy, social care policy, social security policy, agriculture policy, transportation policy, trade policy, etc.[11]

This idea has gradually spread and come to be labeled HiAP over the past quarter-century—and especially over the last decade, most notably in Finland at the turn of this century and then across the European Union (EU) during its Finnish presidency in 2006. In the United States, HiAP was articulated in 2010 by Governor Arnold Schwarzenegger as state policy for California.[12]

The essential ideas of HiAP have also been embodied in proposals since 2009 by the Robert Wood Johnson Foundation and the Obama administration to improve population health and reduce social disparities in health in the United States.[13] These ideas reflect and derive from such efforts in Canada and Europe over the prior decade—most notably a sequel to the earlier Black Report, known as the Acheson Report, which was commissioned and acted upon by the new Labour government of Prime Minister Tony Blair in the final years of the twentieth century.[14]

However, current assessments of implementations and effects of HiAP suggest that at this point it is more rhetoric than reality. Further, in the one instance in which it has been implemented most intensively in terms of spending (£20 billion) and most extensively over time (more than ten years) and space (both nationally and in focal community areas), by the Blair government in the United Kingdom, it failed to achieve its goal of a modest 10 percent reduction of socioeconomic health disparities, which actually increased on some key outcome variables (life expectancy and infant mortality). A careful and thoughtful analysis of the British experience concluded that the reasons lay not in the basic theory of HiAP but in crucial failures in its implementation: (1) the "entry points" and policies were not well chosen in relation to the targeted outcomes; (2) the effects on health were not well enough established a priori; and (3) the scale of implementation, while large, was not adequate to achieve the outcomes desired.[15]

In the British case, and more generally, HiAP has not really been focused on *all* policies, but rather mainly on community-based (as opposed to national) efforts to affect a limited set of health behaviors. Whether through commission or omission, these community interventions have generally failed to address the factors and policies that are most consequential for health, including levels of and disparities in socioeconomic resources and power, as well as problems of discrimination and segregation. And trying to spread the HiAP concept across *all* policies may keep policymakers from carefully and forcefully targeting those policies whose health outcomes would bring the greatest bang for the buck. As we will see, those are likely to be national socioeconomic policies, which may face much greater political resistance than broader, small-scale policies at the local and community level.

This chapter has provided a sense of the potential nature and effects of demand-side health policy, as well as the limitations of current efforts in these directions. Chapters 7 and 8 will focus on the two key issues for any demand-side approach to health and health care expenditure, which must be based on social determinants and disparities in health: What should be the focal social determinants of health for demand-side health policy, and what is the evidence that changes in these can improve population health? And what is the evidence that improving levels of population health and reducing social disparities in health will reduce expenditures on health care and insurance?

Chapter 7

Socioeconomic Policies That Affect Health and Health Disparities

HISTORICALLY, DEMAND-SIDE health policies have been largely grounded in biomedical science. The demand-side approach we need now, however, must focus far more heavily on social determinants and disparities in health. It must identify and prioritize socioeconomic and other public policies that significantly improve individual and population health, reduce health disparities, and feasibly and cost-effectively reduce health care and insurance expenditures.

The health consequences of socioeconomic policies are often not obvious, and typically they are neither anticipated nor recognized at the policymaking stage. In addition, some people have other reasons to resist changes in socioeconomic policies that affect health. Throughout this book, I have argued that we can and must shape socioeconomic policy to promote health and reduce health disparities, thereby reducing health expenditures, and we have already gone some way in achieving this goal. Of course, our continuing efforts should seek to have the greatest positive and least negative effects on other outcomes of our socioeconomic policies—or what economists term "externalities"—whether intended or unintended.

Examples from Past and Present Policy

My wife and I spent the 2010–2011 academic year living in the Upper East Side of New York City, and we got to see and know many areas of Manhattan. What immediately strikes one in Manhattan—at least in the area below the north end of Central Park and Harlem—is that very few people smoke and almost no one is overweight or obese, except for the many tourists in midtown Manhattan. Statistics from population surveys and health data confirm this observational impression.

How did central and lower Manhattan come to look this way, in contrast to many other areas of New York City and, even more so, other areas of the United States? It is partially a story of the benefits of the high levels of education and income that characterize this population. But it is also a story of the often unintended effects of social and economic policies seemingly far removed from health, coupled with targeted public health policies that have been largely socioeconomic rather than biomedical in nature.

Cigarette Smoking

As seen in figure 3.1, cigarette smoking is essentially a twentieth-century phenomenon. The growing of tobacco and its manufacture into cigarettes originally had nothing to do with health. The tobacco industry was an outgrowth of agricultural and economic policies, especially in the Southern United States, that sought to increase economic productivity in developing rural and urban areas. Tobacco was a very profitable cash crop that grew well in the Southern climate and soil, and developments in manufacturing technology made it profitable to dry the tobacco and process it into cigarettes in the factories of cities near the tobacco fields.

When my family lived in Durham, North Carolina, in the early to mid-1970s, the sweet smell of tobacco drying in warehouses permeated the city (and the ballpark of the Durham Bulls, of movie fame). Cigarette company headquarters and manufacturing plants were a mainstay of the economy. Smoking was permitted in all classrooms and offices of Duke University and in almost all areas of the Duke University Medical Center other than where explosive gases were in use. ENJOY SMOKING TOBACCO PRODUCTS bumper stickers emblazoned the cars of many natives and even those of some of the influx of Northerners to the growing Research Triangle. Because taxes on cigarettes were virtually nonexistent, you could buy a carton of cigarettes—and we did—for less than the price of a pack in most places today, certainly including central Manhattan. All the public and private policies and developments that fostered the growing, manufacture, and consumption of tobacco in the early twentieth century, though not intended to harm individual or population health, gave no thought to the health effects of smoking.

However, as also seen in figure 3.1, evidence began to appear in the second quarter of the century that cigarette smoking and other uses of tobacco products were contributing to increasing rates of lung and other respiratory cancers. First noticed by observant clinicians, this impact was documented in larger prospective studies showing that smokers compared to nonsmokers had double the risk of all-cause mortality, a sevenfold greater risk of heart disease, and ten to twenty times the risk of lung and respiratory cancers. These alarming rates were exacerbated in people who were also exposed to environmental hazards such as asbestos and radon. The Surgeon General's report on smoking and health of 1964 began a half-century effort—now quite, though not completely, successful—to reduce cigarette smoking and consequent respiratory disease and cancer as well as heart disease.

In the 1960s and much of the 1970s, many people said that we could not or should not try to deter people from "enjoying tobacco products" or restrain farmers and tobacco companies from producing them. In some senses they were right. Biomedical efforts to clinically convince individuals to stop smoking or chewing tobacco proved largely ineffective. Similarly fruitless were efforts, heavily financed by the tobacco industry, to "detoxify tobacco" to make its use harmless—not to mention efforts to redirect growers and manufacturers away from a highly profitable endeavor.

However, aided greatly by the discovery of the adverse health effects of exposure to secondhand smoke, new kinds of public policy reduced the demand for tobacco products. Probably most important were higher taxes on tobacco products, such that in New York City in 2011 a single pack of cigarettes cost around $15, several times the cost of a carton of ten packs in Durham in the 1970s. More and more restrictions have since been placed on where people can smoke: workplaces, schools, medical institutions, and restaurants were the first to limit and then eliminate smoking, and now even bars and many outside public areas restrict smoking. New York City has been among the most aggressive in pursuing these health-oriented social and economic policies. As a growing antismoking social movement helped to produce these policy changes, smoking became increasingly stigmatized, especially at higher socioeconomic levels. These developments have been the major factors reducing smoking in the United States and Canada and increasingly in Europe. Cigarette consumption and production has shifted to areas of Africa, Asia, and Latin America.[1]

Obesity

Obesity has been replacing smoking as what is viewed as the nation's major public health problem. Widespread obesity is a relatively new phenomenon, though not as de novo as smoking in the early twentieth century. Since the early 1980s, obesity has more than doubled in the United States, and extreme or morbid obesity has increased severalfold. Again, this growing public health problem is largely the outgrowth of social and economic policies that go back a century or more, with little or no consideration of their health effects.

America was for several centuries a nation of farmers, and facilitating the productivity and profitability of American farms has long been a major goal of public policy. This has also served the public health goal of ensuring that the entire population would have an adequate food supply. American agricultural policies, in fostering the production of commodities such as wheat, corn, sugar, soybeans, dairy products, and meat and poultry rather than fruits and vegetables, have helped to make the United States a major food exporter.

More than half of Americans lived and worked on farms even at the beginning of the twentieth century, yet fewer than 3 percent do so today. Farms and agribusiness have become very large and continue to focus on the same commodities, supported by national, state, and local agricultural policies. Unfortunately, many of these commodities are high in calories, sugar, and saturated fats, which we have learned over the past half-century or so contribute to overweight, diabetes, heart disease, and some forms of cancer. Thus, quite unintentionally, well-intended agricultural policy has probably made some contribution to the growing epidemic of chronic disease, and now especially of obesity and diabetes, in American society. Also contributing have been changes in where and how food is prepared and eaten—less often at home and more often in restaurants and, most recently, fast-food outlets. Unfortunately, definitive estimates of the impact of these and other factors are hard to find.[2]

Apart from accidents, farmers have for many years been one of the healthiest occupational groups in the American population, despite heavily consuming the same products and following the same diet on which their agriculture has been focused. Although traditionally their consumption of high levels of calories, sugar, and fats was necessary for the high levels of physical activity involved in farm work, over time farm work has become more mechanized and the levels of physical exertion it requires have diminished. The same has become even more true of work and life in most urban areas. Land use, housing, and transportation in America evolved over the twentieth century as we moved from a primarily rural and agricultural society to a heavily urban and industrialized, now commercialized, nation.

Early in the twentieth century, migrants from rural areas went to major urban centers such as New York City, Chicago, and the other large cities of the Northeast and Midwest. The public health challenges in those cities were sanitation and population density, but not lack of physical activity. Much work at that time was still physically demanding, and to get anywhere, whether to and from work or school or out on the town for the night, people still mainly walked, rode a bicycle, or used a growing system of mass bus and rail transportation (getting to and from which usually required walking). Although most workplaces in cities today are offices or service industry sites like hotels and restaurants, nonwork life in many cities continues to involve walking and public transportation. We lived a year very enjoyably in New York City without a car, walking several miles a day at least several days a week as part of our daily routine—which was very close to the level of physical activity now recommended by public health agencies. Upon returning to Ann Arbor, where we typically need or choose to drive almost everywhere and have to make a conscious decision to walk more than going to or from our cars, we initially resented the degree to which our cars dominated our lives, not only reducing our physical activity but also contributing greatly to air pollution.

The evolution over the twentieth century of metropolitan areas from densely populated central cities where people got around by walking, cycling, or using public rail and bus transportation to much more spread out, lower-density patterns of largely suburban housing, with cars as the main mode of transportation, is the outcome of a century of public policy in the areas of economic and urban development, housing, and transportation: Again, policy made with little regard for health, and certainly with no conception or anticipation of adverse health effects. Economic, urban development, and housing policies fostered the growth of owner-occupied single-family homes, by necessity in the suburbs of major central cities, in contrast to the patterns of denser rental housing that characterized the cities. These housing policies were supported and even encouraged by economic, urban development, and transportation policies based on the movement of people via cars and goods via trucks. Funding for roads and bridges—and later for airports to facilitate long-distance travel—came to dominate and crowd out funding for rail and other forms of mass transportation. Our systems of urban freeways and interstate highways are the most obvious manifestations of these policies.[3]

Thus, again quite inadvertently, people have become sedentary in their work and leisure, while agricultural and food production and distribution policies continue to generate a quantity and quality of food suited for a decidedly more active population. Fast food—much of which is high in sugar, fat, and salt—and high-caloric soft drinks may be the more proximal contributors to American's obesity epidemic, but they are the logical extensions of much broader and longer-term agriculture, housing, transportation, and urban and economic development policies. Living a year in central Manhattan much as our predecessors did a century ago made all of this much clearer to me.

The health impacts of these nonhealth policies have been exacerbated by policies in education, income, employment, civil rights, and neighborhoods that segregate many urbanites into poor, often minority areas where they have little ability to live the relatively healthful lifestyle of those who, like my family in 2011, are fortunate enough to be able to live and work in central and lower Manhattan. We turn now to this range of other social and economic policies whose health impacts must be considered if we are to improve population health.

Toward Socioeconomic Policy as Health Policy

Smoking and obesity demonstrate the complex and broad web of causation, largely social and economic in nature, that underlies many major health problems. In the case of smoking reduction, we also see the major role that social and economic policies played in producing what is arguably the single greatest public health success of the late twentieth century. We are now searching for analogous levers to arrest and roll back what has been termed the "obesity epidemic." However, we must move beyond responding to specific health and health behavior problems only after they have become severe. We need to identify social and economic policies that can promote health in broad and pervasive ways and thus reduce the need and demand for health care. A growing body of evidence suggests a range of social and economic policies that can have such positive effects on health.

Several criteria are critical to consider when identifying areas of social and economic policy that could be central to a new demand-side health policy. Ideally, we are seeking (1) major established areas of social and economic policy that (2) show broad evidence of causal impacts on a wide range of health outcomes. Such policy should be (3) feasible in terms of technology and resources, (4) cost-effective in the value of its health outcomes relative to its cost, and (5) likely to have other positive effects beyond health and few negative externalities or side effects. Finally, (6) the policy should be politically feasible or palatable, as well as technically possible and promising, though these conditions may only come about with time and struggle, as in the case of antismoking policy. More will be said about these criteria as we consider specific policies.

With smoking and obesity, we have seen that a wide range of policies in which health considerations play some policy role (and could play an even greater role) can be relevant to health, including agricultural, environmental, transportation, and land use policies. In the increasingly global context of health, the impacts of international policies such as diplomacy, defense, immigration, and trade are also relevant and beginning to receive some attention. This chapter highlights five other major and currently debated areas of policy—education policy, income policy, macroeconomic and employment policy, civil rights policy, and housing and neighborhood policy—in which sizable health implications are becoming clearer and could be even greater than we realize.[4] Before turning to these, we should consider the role and nature of scientific evidence in public policy formation regarding health, or any other policy area.

Scientific Evidence and Public Policy

Historically, public policy formation was a function of philosophy more than of science. The chief of staff of a major congressional committee, himself a social scientist and now a member of a major Washington social and economic think tank, once admonished a meeting of social scientists that I attended: "The first thing you need to know is that the main determinants of congressional legislation are the values of the committee chairs." This caveat accords with academic analyses of the policy process, one of which sees three streams converging to create major policy change: a "problem" stream, a "political" stream, and a "policy" stream. That is, any major policy change requires: (1) a widely shared sense that there is a problem that needs to be addressed by policy; (2) a window of time when those with political will are able to enact policy; and (3) reasonable consensus on what kind of policy is needed and is likely to be effective in addressing the perceived problem.[5]

Awareness of health and health care as major problems for American society has crystallized in various ways and times. Most frequently, this awareness has centered on the need to ensure widespread access to medical care. In the 1960s, a skilled and persuasive president with a large political majority (Lyndon Johnson) converged with the clear sense of a need and a way to ensure access to care for the elderly and the poor to produce Medicare and Medicaid. Over the 1970s and 1980s, increases in public and private expenditures for health care and insurance led to growing concerns and efforts to control these expenditures. These concerns were joined in the 1990s by a renewed sense of the lack of adequate or secure medical insurance for the non-elderly population, especially in bad economic times, motivating a new push for national health care reform. But the president (Bill Clinton)—and first lady (Hillary Rodham Clinton)—were unable to galvanize the potential and necessary political and congressional support, owing in part to the lack of a clear consensus on what was the right policy option.

In the 1960s, health care researchers and major political constituencies, from doctors to insurers, had generally seen national health insurance as the only way to effectively provide health insurance for the elderly and needy, who were not profitable for private insurers. In the 1990s, however, views and evidence about how to best insure working people and their families ranged from single-payer national health insurance to various options building on the widespread employer-based insurance system.

The political window opened again in 2009, and the president (Barack Obama) supported congressional leaders who fashioned and ultimately passed in 2010 the Affordable Care Act (ACA), the most comprehensive health care reform since the birth of Medicare and Medicaid. Still, dissension as to the best way to proceed, coupled with political opposition, compromised the breadth and depth of the ACA reform, which continues to be hampered by these forces, even after it narrowly escaped death at the hands of the Supreme Court.[6]

As with past and continuing debates regarding our largely supply-side health care and insurance policies, the role of scientific evidence and policy advocacy is to create clear and relatively consensual policy options that can be accessed when the problem and the political streams converge to create an opportunity for policy change. This book seeks to articulate demand-side options, supported by scientific evidence, in the hope that a wider recognition of our clear and continuing paradoxical crisis of health and health care will soon align with the political willingness and ability to develop and enact a demand-side approach as an essential complement to the current preoccupation with supply-side health care and insurance policies.

Thus, scientific evidence regarding the health impact of nonhealth policies is a sine qua non for identifying and implementing new demand-side approaches to health policy. However, one danger in this—as in any policy area—is that the nature of the evidence seemingly required to move ahead with policy, even in pilot and experimental ways, can be immobilizing, particularly with respect to a crucial causal issue: whether a given policy will have a given effect. For example, can a given area of nonhealth policy improve health and lessen disparities, thereby reducing the need and demand for care and hence expenditures for health care and insurance?

Although all policy is made with less than perfect information regarding the strength, breadth, and causes of the effects of policy, we still want the most and the best evidence we can get. To do so, we must take account of the widest array of evidence—quantitative and qualitative evidence, observational and experimental evidence, and evidence drawn from small and focused populations as well as from large and representative populations. It is the cumulative weight of such evidence—especially the replication and triangulation of results from multiple studies and methods, not any single critical study, experiment, or trial—that supports policy change.

Some argue that only experimental evidence, such as that from randomized clinical trials in medical research, can justify scientific inference and policy action. The less-than-optimal state of current health care practice, even when derived from clinical trials, clearly belies the superiority of experimentation over all other evidence. Trials and experiments can never be carried out on broad and varied enough populations over long enough periods of time to confirm whether some types of people may be adversely (or positively, or just differently) affected by a drug or procedure, or whether similar variations in outcomes will appear over longer time periods than can be studied in clinical trials or experiments. Remember that much highly effective health policy, including antismoking and environmental pollution policy, was necessarily enacted without experimental studies, at least on humans, for whom randomized assignment to exposure to smoking or environmental toxins would be unfeasible and unethical. Experiments and other types of studies are very valuable, especially in conjunction with other evidence, but none are in and of themselves either necessary or sufficient to derive the broad scientific inferences required for major public policy decisions and choices. A large body of convergent evidence across studies and methods not only is necessary but also can be sufficient.[7]

An Exemplary Policy: Education

Probably more than any other area of social policy, education meets, indeed exemplifies, all of the six criteria that are central to formulating demand-side approaches to social policy. From the earliest years of the American nation, education, largely supported by local, state, and federal governments, has been a critical area of public policy because of its role in enabling an informed and effective citizenry. Over time the economic importance of education to both individuals and societies has justified continued and increased investment in it by individuals, families, religious and other nonprofit groups, corporations, and especially governments at all levels.

The United States spends more per student than any nation in the world: about $15,000 per student at all levels in 2010. Across levels of education, we far exceed all nations at the postsecondary level, but rank fourth at the primary and secondary levels (after Luxembourg, Norway, and Switzerland). In terms of education spending as a percentage of gross domestic product, at 7.3 percent in 2010 the United States was tied for sixth with New Zealand among Organization for Economic Cooperation and Development nations (below Denmark, Iceland, Korea, Norway, and Israel). Education is the third-largest area of expenditure by government at all levels, exceeding national defense and surpassed only by pensions and by health care and insurance.

Education policy has received increasing attention in recent years, largely because of problems similar to those of the health care system. For example, despite spending more per student than any nation in the world, the United States now lags behind other nations in years of education completed and in skills acquired in areas such as reading and math.[8] In all of the focus on better measuring the outcomes of education spending, however, almost no attention has been paid to its effects on health.

As we saw in chapter 4, level of education powerfully and pervasively predicts levels of almost all health outcomes—including mortality, morbidity, physical and cognitive functioning, and mental health—as well as almost all risk factors for health. Education is especially important in preventing, or postponing, the onset of health problems. Further, studies, especially over the past decade, have documented educational disparities in health in the United States (see figure 4.2). The vast preponderance of evidence indicates that increasing years of education *causes* increasing levels of health, both within and across nations.[9]

Even cross-sectional correlations between years of education and health in middle or older age are putatively causal because formal education is completed by age eighteen for many people, and by age twenty-five to thirty or so for almost all. Educational attainment clearly precedes adult health, though both can be affected by childhood health. More compelling are the many prospective or longitudinal studies in which years of education predicts subsequent health outcomes, after adjusting for levels of health at the start of the observation period and with education levels fixed at the onset of the study.

For those who still worry that some factor not observed or controlled at the beginning of the prospective study (such as genes) may be producing the association between health and education, both quasi-experimental and experimental evidence also consistently indicate that increasing years of education leads to improvements in health. For example, multiple studies show that when states or nations have raised the number of years of compulsory schooling, the people who were first affected by the change lived longer than the individuals who completed school under the prior compulsory schooling policy. Finally, a number of evaluation studies have randomly assigned children to receive more or better early childhood education. The studies that have evaluated childhood and adult health outcomes generally find significantly better health among those randomly allocated to receive more or better early childhood education compared to those who were randomly allocated not to receive it.

Thus, simply increasing the number of years of education people receive, not to mention improving its quality, can significantly improve their health. This can be done in a variety of ways, including increased financial support. One study showed that each $10,000 of additional financial aid to a postsecondary student (in 1998 dollars) results on average in 1.6 more years of post–high school education. This in turn can result in 0.3 to 1.0 additional years of life. Economists would minimally value these additional years of life at $20,000 to $75,000. Thus, the $10,000 investment in education has a 200 to 750 percent rate of return in the economic value of its health effects.

Since education has even stronger effects on health than on mortality, increasing education is likely also to reduce the need for and utilization of health care. Thus, investments in education can be highly cost-effective in improving health—much more so than many forms of preventive or therapeutic health care. For example, whereas the $10,000 investment in education buys up to one year of life, estimates in 2008 indicated that the average cost of lifetime medical spending for a year's increase in life expectancy ranged over the life course from $30,000 to $145,000 for the period 1990 to 2000. In other words, at best, health care is dollar for dollar no more effective than education in improving life expectancy, and at worst, at least several times *less* effective than education.[10]

We still have a great deal to learn about exactly how and why level of education improves health. Figure 7.1 shows the marginal effects of each year of education for age zero through seventeen and older on a range of health and health behaviors in the National Health Interview Survey. The marginal effects are essentially the difference in the predicted probability of an outcome at a given level of education compared to the average predicted probability (or scale score for depression) in the population, adjusting for the effects of race and gender. The important point of the graph is to show whether the levels of a given outcome increase or decrease as years of education increase.

It is clear that the impact of education varies across health outcomes, with larger effects on health than on longevity. It is also clear that for some variables (for example, fair or poor health, any functional limitations, depression), individuals receive additional health benefits from graduating from high school or graduating from college (beyond just another year of education). Further, it is clear that the effects of education on health may begin operating even before schooling is complete, as evidenced in the strong effects of education, especially high school completion, on some health behaviors (for example, smoking and seat belt use).

Finally, although we know that the impact of education on health and health risk factors varies over time, age, place, and other factors, most notably declining in older age, it is almost always consequential. Education's effects on health may be due to its effect on occupation and income and wealth attainment (discussed in the next section), on health behaviors, and on access to and more effective use of new medical technology, or its effects may be due to other factors. Learning more about the pathways and mechanisms through which education affects health can help to develop more effectively targeted educational policies for improving health. But it is already clear that simply increasing years of educational attainment, and especially completing high school and college, can substantially improve health, thus reducing the need and demand for health care. It follows that: (1) we should evaluate the health effects of any major educational policy or intervention; (2) we should factor the health effects of education into any cost-benefit analysis of both health policy and education policy; and (3) we should make investments in education part of a new demand-side policy for improving population health and reducing health care expenditures.

Figure 7.1 The Effects of Education on Various Health Measures, by Single Year of Schooling

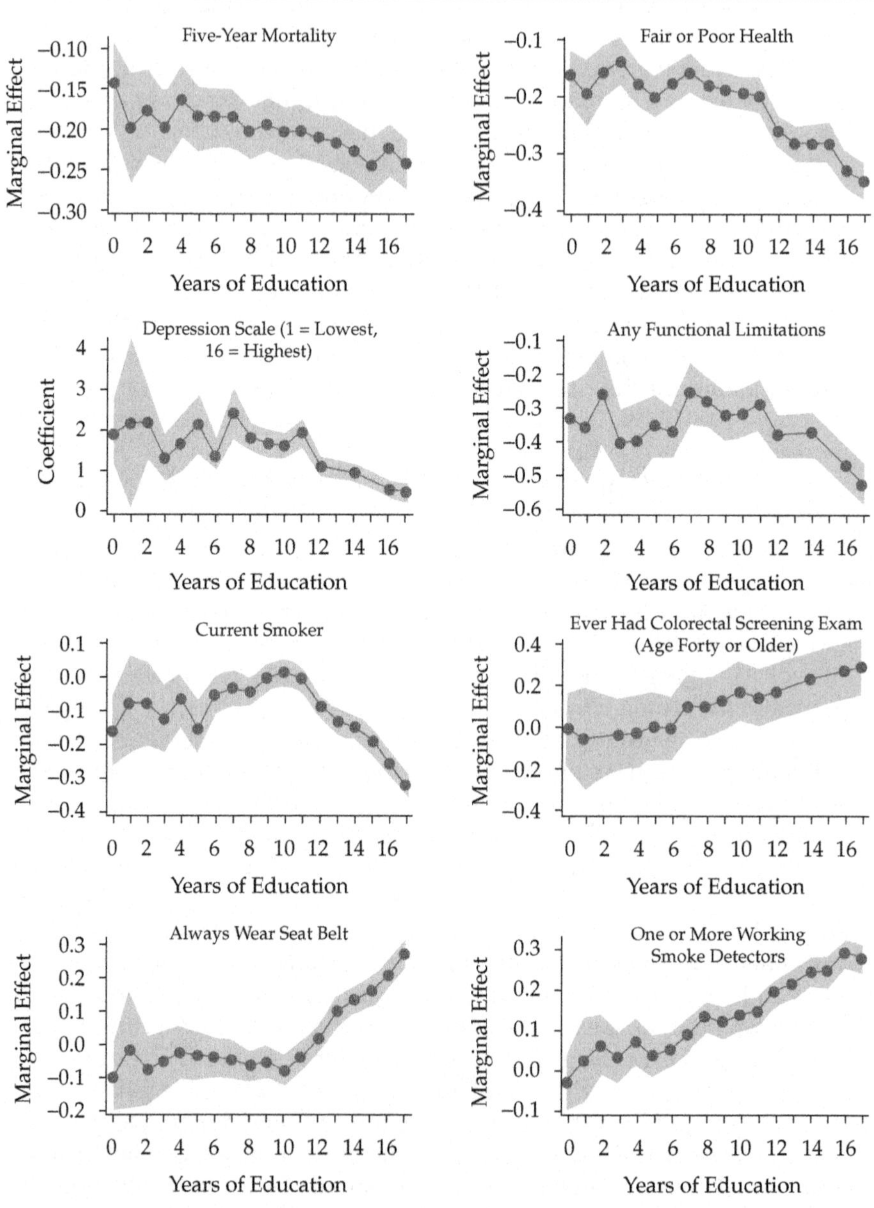

Source: Schoeni et al. (2008, figure 2.2).
Note: Marginal effects from logit regressions on education, controlling for race and gender. The shaded areas are 95 percent confidence levels for each coefficient. See text for explanation of marginal effects.

The many other positive effects or externalities of increased education, such as improved jobs and incomes and enhanced labor force productivity, make education economically and politically attractive as a lever for also improving health. Initial estimates suggest that the health benefit of education could represent up to a 50 percent increase in the returns to education that individuals currently receive via higher occupational attainment and earnings.[11] Given that we already spend about $1 trillion on education, the marginal increment for new expenditures would be modest and the returns high in terms of health as well as other benefits. Conversely, constraining or reducing many types of expenditures for education is likely only to exacerbate our paradoxical crisis of spending more and more for health care and insurance yet having a less healthy population. As we will see in chapter 9, reductions in some areas of support for education have probably already done so.

Income Policies and Health

Unlike education, the idea that government and public policy have a responsibility to support and ensure the incomes of the American people does not go back to the founding decades of our nation. However, as America transitioned from a rural and agricultural society to an urban and industrial one in the nineteenth and twentieth centuries, government, in conjunction with private employers, began to assume a role in supporting the incomes of those unable to earn at least subsistence-level incomes owing to disability, job loss, old age, and, more recently, insufficient earnings even when working full-time in the paid labor force. The biggest portion of this support is through pensions, especially Old-Age, Survivors, and Disability Insurance (OASDI) commonly known as Social Security. As a proportion of GDP, pension spending is second only to health and health care; in 2009, it accounted for over 9.7 percent of U.S. GDP, of which 6.8 percent was government spending.[12]

Spending on pensions at all levels of government and in the private sector has become a focus of political and policy discussion, with no clear resolution yet in sight. Concerns about pension expenditures have been extended to other programs designed to provide income support to those unable to work or to earn a minimally sufficient income (defined as 100 to 200 percent of the poverty level), from welfare to food stamps, unemployment and disability insurance, the minimum wage, and the Earned Income Tax Credit (EITC). In all the discussions about reducing (or expanding) these programs, almost no attention has been paid to their consequences for health.

As with education, a great deal of evidence has led to a widespread recognition of the association or correlation between income and health. In contrast to education, however, it seems much more possible, or even plausible, that adult health affects adult income, as well as vice versa. Thus, it is reassuring that almost all studies using income at a given point in life to predict health over many years thereafter have found that income is usually at least as strong a predictor of future health as education, if not stronger. Income is less important than education in preventing or postponing the onset of health problems, but much more important in slowing the progression of health problems and delaying mortality. Health also predicts income, though usually over much shorter periods, as when an illness or decline in health reduces earnings or depletes savings for a few weeks to a few years.[13]

A growing body of intriguing and important experimental and quasi-experimental evidence has also been generated over the past ten to twenty years. Multiple studies have found sizable impacts on health from changes in income support policies, as well as from other exogenous "shocks" to income that could not be the products of individuals' health. The kinds of exogenous shocks examined have included lottery winnings, changes in income due to the reunification of East and West Germany, increases in food stamp allocations, and changes in levels of payment via income support programs such as the EITC and Supplemental Security Income (SSI, for persons with disability and for elderly people with poverty-level incomes even after Social Security payments).[14]

Nationally, the largest and most effective income support program has been Social Security, created in the late 1930s as part of the New Deal and indexed to inflation in the 1960s and early 1970s. Social Security has been the most effective antipoverty program in our nation's history. It reduced poverty among the elderly from over 40 percent prior to its inception and greater than 20 percent even after its inception but before benefits were indexed to inflation to less than 10 percent in recent decades—the lowest poverty level of any age group in the population. Because from the outset it was a universal national program, and also because it has coincided with major advances in medical practice, such as antibiotics (from the 1940s onward) and health insurance (Medicare), it is impossible to establish a clear causal impact of Social Security on health. It is highly suggestive, however, that today the United States compares most favorably to other developed countries on a variety of health indicators among the elderly, and further, that improvements in the health of the elderly have been most marked in the periods following the inception of Social Security (1940–1955) and then following the indexing of Social Security to inflation (1970–1985). The health of the elderly improved during these periods both relative to rates of improvement in the health of the elderly in prior decades and relative to improvement in the health of people younger than sixty-five, as can be seen in figure 7.2.[15]

Other research has demonstrated that exogenous changes in SSI for the poor elderly have positive impacts on their health. An initial study

Figure 7.2 Mortality Trends and the Implementation of Social Security, 1900–1995

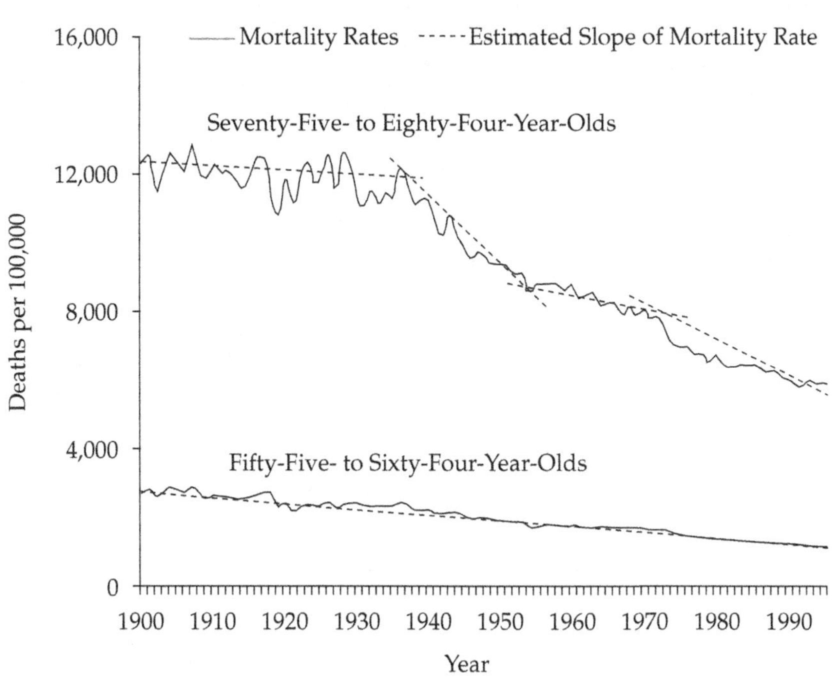

Source: Schoeni et al. (2008, figure 4.1).

showed that the original introduction of SSI benefits eliminated a preexisting difference in health between those eligible for SSI and the more affluent elderly. A later study focused on variation over time in state supplements to federal SSI payments. Each $100-per-month increase in SSI predicted a 1.8-percentage-point decline (for example, from 38 percent to 36.2 percent) in the disability rate among the elderly in the bottom quartile of the income distribution. An increase of $500 per month would reduce disability by almost 10 percentage points—again, a very positive rate of return.[16]

Finally, Latin American countries, beginning with Mexico, have implemented large income support programs for the poor over the last two decades, with the goal of improving child and family health. Usually referred to as conditional cash transfer programs, they provide income supplements to the poor, usually on the condition that they ensure that their children receive preventive medical care and attend primary school. The programs have been randomly introduced over time into poor villages, creating an experimental comparison of villages that received benefits earlier with ones that did not receive them until later. Results show positive impacts on child health as well as on the health of mothers and other family members. The relative importance for health outcomes of the added income versus the required health and education behaviors remains to be precisely determined. However, studies in Ecuador, where income supports were initially provided unconditionally, clearly show that even income alone produces substantial health benefits. The positive health effects of income support have also been seen in evaluations of the introduction of old-age pensions for blacks in post-apartheid South Africa.[17]

Thus, we have strong evidence that public policies providing income supports to needy portions of the population can also have substantial positive impacts on their health. These health effects need to be accounted for in any analysis of the costs and benefits of increasing or reducing income supports, issues which are at the center of current policy debates about how to control our burgeoning health care expenditures and debt levels more generally. Further, we need to better assess and quantify both the health benefits of income support policies and their implications for health care and insurance utilization and expenditures. Like education policy, income support policies may be as cost-effective for improving health as major traditional health care and insurance policies and practices, if not more so; in the process, they may also reduce the need and expenditures for health care and insurance. Also as with education, reductions in the income support programs discussed here are likely to only exacerbate our paradoxical crisis of declining population health despite growing expenditures on health care and insurance. Since we already spend over $1 trillion on income support programs, the marginal cost of new expenditures would necessarily be modest.

Macroeconomic, Monetary, and Fiscal Policy

Although it represents nowhere near as large a fraction of GDP or government spending as education and income policy, in either the public or private sector, macroeconomic policy in both its fiscal and monetary aspects is one of the most central responsibilities and activities of the federal government. Indeed, since 2008 macroeconomic policy has arguably been the central preoccupation of our government and politics, as it has historically tended to be in periods of either recession and unemployment or hyperexpansion and inflation. Again, however, this preoccupation has included little or no consideration of the impact of macroeconomic cycles and policies on health or on expenditures for health care and insurance.

One of the great achievements of social science and public policy between the Great Depression and the Great Recession was to develop a considerable degree of consensus on how fiscal (spending) policies and monetary (interest and credit) policies combine, in both the private sphere and especially the public sphere, to affect the growth of the economy and related levels of employment and inflation. The overall goal of macroeconomic policy is to maintain substantially positive rates of economic growth and low rates of unemployment (both in the 3 to 5 percent range) while also maintaining modestly low levels of inflation (around 2 percent) so that, on balance, there is sustained and steady growth of real economic output and income, and hence societal and individual well-being. However, it is far easier and more politically palatable to enact fiscal and monetary policies to counteract recessionary tendencies—by increasing public and private spending through lower taxes and deficit spending or increasing the money supply by lowering interest rates and essentially printing new money (quantitative easing)—than it is to enact policies to counteract excessive economic growth and employment—for example, reducing private and public spending through higher taxes and budget cuts or decreasing the money supply through higher interest rates.

As with other nonhealth policies, the health impacts of macroeconomic cycles and policies are substantial but largely unrecognized—in this case partly because they are fundamentally paradoxical. Reasonably well established and recognized are the adverse effects on both socioeconomic well-being and health that accrue to individuals experiencing unemployment and declining income and socioeconomic position as a result of economic contractions or recessions. Perhaps most striking, among middle-aged workers with substantial job tenure, job loss due to a major economic recession can result in a lifetime loss of $10,000 to $15,000 per year in income and one and a half years of life expectancy, with income loss probably the major mediator of the effects of job loss on mortality.[18]

Modern macroeconomic policy includes actions to buffer the impact of economic recession on individuals who experience job or income loss. Unemployment benefits, food stamps, and other programs more or less automatically kick in to counteract the adverse consequences of an economic downturn, though the level and length of receipt of such benefits tends to be lower in the United States than in other comparably wealthy nations. To the extent that these programs (or private ones such as employer or union economic support or other household members increasing their income) mitigate the economic losses associated with job loss, they also mitigate the health effects. These expenditures also provide a fiscal stimulus toward renewed economic growth. Thus, strengthening such programs can provide major returns in alleviating health problems as well as stimulating economic demand and hence output.

Paradoxically, evidence also indicates that mortality and most health

Figure 7.3 Life Expectancy at Birth, Unemployment Rate, and Economic Growth in the United States, 1920–1940

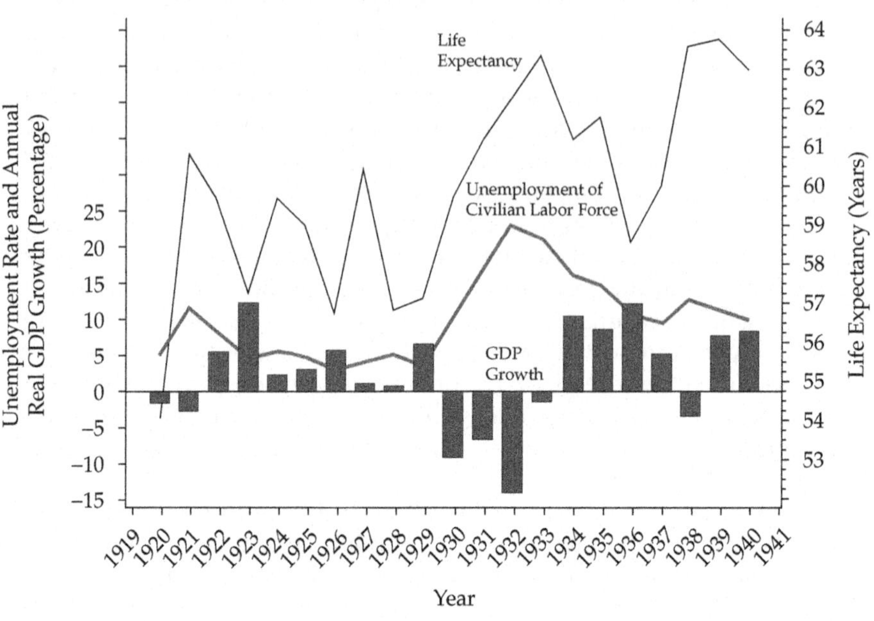

Source: Tapia Granados and Diez Roux (2009, figure 1).

problems (except suicide) vary procyclically with the state of the economy. That is, net of overall trends over time (for example, the general improvement in health and decline in mortality for the last 250 years or so), overall population health actually declines during economic expansions and improves during economic recessions and even depressions. This was true even for the Great Depression, as shown in figure 7.3.[19]

What could explain why *population* health improves during recessions when many *individuals* are experiencing job or income loss and consequent adverse health effects? And why does population health worsen during economic expansions, when fewer individuals suffer job and income loss and the job and income situations of many are improving? The answer appears to be that only a minority of the population (25 percent or fewer even in the Great Depression) are experiencing job or income loss at any point during an economic contraction, while the entire population is subjected to increased health risks from a variety of correlates or consequences of economic expansion. Most clearly and notably, traffic accidents and fatalities rise by 10 percent or so during expansions because people drive more, and they decline comparably during recessions, when people drive less. Similarly, greater employment and work activity increases the rate of accidental injury and death at work. Increased economic activity also increases levels of pollution and environmental hazards, as well as working time and stress, while reducing time for leisure, physical, and other recreational activity. Health behaviors such as eating, drinking, and smoking also worsen during economic expansions because people can better afford to smoke, drink, and overeat; conversely, these behaviors improve during economic downturns, when people are less able to afford their bad habits. Since all of these changes affect most or all of the population, for the total population during a recession these salutary effects outweigh the quite adverse health effects among the minority of individuals who lose jobs or incomes. Changes of 3 to 5 percent in unemployment rates—the levels that characterize shifts from economic recession to economic expansion—produce changes in health that approximate those associated with one and a half to two and a half years of aging.[20]

These broader adverse health effects of economic growth are not currently addressed at all in socioeconomic or health policy. They certainly could be addressed, however, using policies that would also have the kind of spending reduction effects needed to avoid excessive rates of inflation. We currently tax in various ways most of the behaviors and activities that contribute to increased mortality and morbidity in times of economic growth—for example, excise taxes on cigarettes and alcohol, fuel taxes, and taxes on pollution emissions. These could be extended to high-calorie foods. Further, if such taxes were indexed to economic growth, they could rise during economic expansions, thus mitigating their adverse health consequences while also serving to moderate the rate of economic expansion to keep it at non-inflationary levels. Conversely, indexed taxes could automatically be reduced during times of economic contraction, returning money to consumers, who could then increase their spending in ways that should be no worse for their health than their spending before the recession. The effect could even be health-enhancing if they shifted some or all of their savings on cigarettes, alcohol, high-calorie food, and gasoline toward healthier or at least more neutral choices.[21]

Thus, macroeconomic policy could have substantial positive impacts on health via taxation and income support policies that would also help to restore and sustain the primary purpose of macroeconomic policy—steady economic and employment growth with low inflation. As with education and income policies, considering and measuring health effects should become a more central component of macroeconomic policy, just as macroeconomic policy should be a key component of health policy.

Civil Rights Policy and Health

Like macroeconomic policy, the development and implementation of civil rights policy is a major focus of politics and government but not in itself a major aspect of economic activity in either the public or private sector. And like macroeconomic policy, civil rights policy has major implications for health, the extent of which has only recently been recognized. Thus, beyond issues of equal access to health care, health has not yet played a significant role in the thinking about either civil rights policy or health policy. Civil rights policy focuses on achieving equality of opportunity and, by implication, equality of results in political, social, and economic realms across groups that differ in ways, largely physical and cultural, that do not preclude such equality. Because of the magnitude and nature of the inequalities that civil rights policy seeks to overcome, the outcomes of such policy, including health outcomes, have always been quite variable and complex.

The nineteenth and twentieth centuries in America and around the world have seen major transformations in civil rights policies and hence the social opportunities and standings of various groups. Mainly this has involved change from national and international social orders dominated by whites (over people of color) and men (over women) toward societies with more equal opportunity and results across gender and racial-ethnic groups. Though these changes have been large to date, they are also still incomplete in ways that are important in terms of both sociopolitics and health.

Race-Ethnicity and the Civil Rights Movement

Arguably, the scope of change in this country has been greatest in terms of race-ethnicity, especially for African Americans. Over the course of American history, but especially since World War II, the status of African Americans has moved from a legally segregated and inferior caste to increasingly equal members of society. Although legally sanctioned segregation, discrimination, and inferior social position were essentially abolished de jure by the Civil Rights Acts of the 1960s, that abolition is not yet fully de facto. More and more evidence suggests that the breakdown of legal discrimination in all areas of life has profoundly improved the sociopolitical status, and hence health, of African Americans. However, the persistence of de facto segregation and discrimination—especially in housing and hence also schools, job opportunities, health care, and socioeconomic position—continues to adversely affect the health of racial-ethnic minorities.

The dramatic dismantling in the 1950s and 1960s of de jure segregation and discrimination against African Americans, especially in the South, had large and pervasive beneficial impacts on their socioeconomic opportunities and attainment, as well as their access to medical care, with related improvements in health. Again especially in the South, when African Americans were granted equal access to hospitals and other health care facilities, the improvements in infant and maternal mortality were dramatic.[22] Socioeconomically, African American women, again especially in the South, were liberated from employment largely as domestic servants and began to work in clerical, sales, and even professional and technical jobs, often in the public sector, with resulting improvements in their working conditions and income. In 1964, over half of all African American women age thirty-eight to sixty-five in the South were employed as domestic servants, as were about one-third of African American women outside the South. By 1980, these rates were under 20 percent in the South and under 10 percent outside the South. Over the same period, the percentage of African American women in the South employed in white-collar occupations rose from 10 percent to 20 percent (and from 20 percent to 50 percent outside the South). In some age groups, these changes virtually equalized the incomes of black and white women; blacks had earned a full one-third less than whites prior to implementation of the civil rights laws.[23]

With a slight lag, the greatest progress in reducing mortality and increasing life expectancy during the late 1960s and 1970s was made among African American women, especially in the South but also in other regions, as shown in figure 7.4. Years of increase in the life expectancy of black women more than tripled in the 1965–1974 decade over the 1955–1964 decade, again especially in the South. These gains outstripped those of black men, as well as whites, none of whom experienced occupational and economic gains as great as those of black women.

Although it is highly plausible that these health improvements derived from the civil rights policies enacted in the 1960s and 1970s, the evidence comes largely from comparing over-time changes in occupations, income, and health. There is as yet little direct evidence at the individual level, and there is certainly no experimental data. The results are quite consistent, however, with quasi-experimental results on the health impacts of improved socioeconomic opportunities for blacks in post-apartheid South Africa.[24] Further, these results are congruent with ingenious new research showing that court-ordered school desegregation in the South and North in the 1960s and 1970s—the timing of which across school districts was quasi-random—had very sizable positive impacts on the subsequent socioeconomic attainment and health of black children over their adult lives. It should be noted that these effects were driven

Figure 7.4 Change in Life Expectancy at Age Thirty-Five in the United States, 1955–1964 and 1965–1974

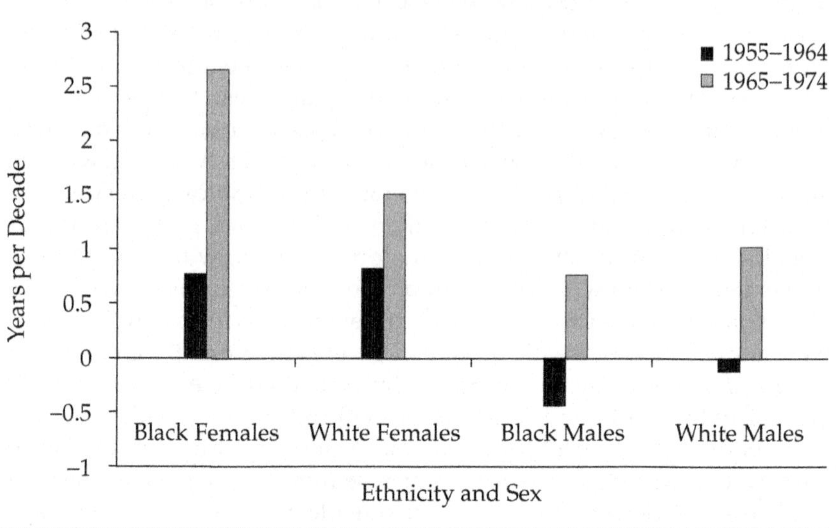

Source: Schoeni et al. (2008, figure 6.7).

largely by improved funding of predominantly black schools in the South and North and secondarily by the effects of more blacks attending schools with whites.[25]

Despite all these positive effects of de jure equalization of the positions of whites and blacks and blacks' consequent access to better education, occupations, and incomes, blacks on average remain de facto segregated and unequal in terms of housing, schools, and jobs, as well as in the quality of the health care they receive, even with no apparent legal barriers to access.[26] This appears to reflect persisting de facto or "institutional" discrimination, which can limit opportunities without clear overt discrimination. For example, a variety of housing, economic, and job policies and trends make it more likely that blacks will be concentrated in areas with poorer access to quality housing and schools, good public services, socioeconomic resources, healthful living conditions, and even medical care.[27] Evidence suggests that this segregation and the stress levels associated with it explain a significant portion of the persisting racial differences in health.

For example, despite quite successful efforts to eliminate racial differences in awareness and treatment of high blood pressure, blacks continue to be more likely to have high blood pressure and to be less likely to have their blood pressure controlled by treatment. The persisting differences in prevalence disappear when blacks and whites are statistically equalized in terms of their neighborhood conditions and their anticipation of stress in daily life. The blood pressure of blacks also may increase if they are constantly anticipating either legal discrimination (such as in jobs or housing) or everyday discrimination (being treated less well than others). The racial difference in blood pressure disappears if blacks and whites report being equally vigilant against discrimination (on the basis of age, gender, or other things as well as race).[28]

In sum, evidence suggests that civil rights policies that equalize opportunities for and attainment of better conditions of life and work can markedly improve the health of racial-ethnic minorities. Similarly, failure to fully equalize such opportunities may help to explain persisting racial-ethnic disparities in health. Parallel, though very preliminary, findings are beginning to appear in relation to the effects of policies equalizing such opportunities and attainments for nonheterosexual portions of our population. All indications are that civil rights policy remains a potent mechanism for improving health and reducing health disparities and, in turn, the need for, utilization of, and spending for health care. Again, consideration and assessment of health must become part of all civil rights policy formation, and civil rights policy should become more central to health policy.

Changing Gender Disparities in Health

The lack of full and comprehensive implementation of civil rights policies with respect to race-ethnicity has constrained improvements in minorities' opportunities and attainment in the socioeconomic and health realms. As noted in chapter 5, it is possible that the large (if also incomplete) gains in opportunities and achievements for women in the educational and occupational realms have both produced and increased exposure to some health risks, such as smoking and occupational injury and illness. Combined with a lack of commensurate equalization of rights and responsibilities in the sphere of family life, these socioeconomic gains may be creating adverse effects on women's health and a declining female advantage over men in mortality and life expectancy. Civil rights and other social policies that make the gender revolution more complete might reverse these potential and unanticipated adverse effects of civil rights advances in the occupational sphere.

Housing and Neighborhood Policy

This chapter began by noting that housing and neighborhood policy in the United States has historically supported a rural agricultural economy and homeownership, even as the country has become increasingly urban and industrialized. These policies, along with transportation policies favoring automobiles and airplanes over railroads and urban mass transit, have contributed to the growing obesity "epidemic" in our society, although the contribution of housing and transportation policies has yet to be well estimated, either absolutely or relative to other policies. More recently, however, there has been increasing interest in the contribution of the nature of social contexts, communities, and neighborhoods to health and health problems.

To the extent that the Obama administration has attended to social determinants of health outside of the Affordable Care Act, this attention has been mainly focused within the Department of Housing and Urban Development and its Healthy Communities initiatives. Similarly, the major private initiative to extend the focus of health policy beyond health care and insurance, the Robert Wood Johnson Foundation Commission to Build a Healthier America, made creating "Healthier Homes and Communities" one of its central foci and recommendations, along with improving health behaviors and promoting child health and development. Evidence suggests that neighborhoods and social contexts may be consequential factors in health. That evidence, however, is generally more limited and localized than the evidence for the health impacts of the other policy areas we have considered. And housing and neighborhoods represent a relatively new and modest-sized area of social policy.

A growing body of evidence, mostly from studies of individual cities and communities and a small number of national studies, finds that people living in socioeconomically disadvantaged neighborhoods have poorer health than those living in more advantaged ones, over and above the effects of individuals' socioeconomic levels. That is, living in a disadvantaged neighborhood constitutes a risk factor for health in addition to the high risk associated with being poor, and living in a neighborhood inhabited mainly by highly educated people has health benefits beyond those attributable to a person's own level of education.

The precise aspects of neighborhoods that produce these effects, the health outcomes most affected, and the mechanisms or processes connecting neighborhoods to health are less well understood. The lack of places and contexts for purchasing good food or engaging in physical activities appears to play some role, as do exposure to environmental hazards and pollutants and the stresses induced by fear of crime, noise, and so forth. As noted in relation to civil rights, the segregation of blacks into neighborhoods with disadvantaged and stressful living conditions may explain much of the persisting higher levels of hypertension in blacks relative to whites.[29]

Available evidence comes largely from studies at one point in time, in contrast to the growing body of longitudinal and time series studies linking the prior policy areas we have considered to health. And experimental evidence has been almost entirely lacking until recently. The Moving to Opportunity (MTO) program of the U.S. Department of Housing and Urban Development randomly assigned residents of public housing in five cities to three conditions: (1) receiving traditional (Section 8) housing vouchers to subsidize rent and enable them to move to private and presumably better housing; (2) receiving the same vouchers with associated requirements and assistance in moving to a clearly less poor neighborhood (less than 10 percent of residents in poverty); or (3) simply remaining in public housing. The original MTO experiment was focused on educational and labor market outcomes for children and adults, but the initial five-year evaluation suggested possible beneficial effects on health as well. Health outcomes were addressed more extensively in the ten-year evaluation, which produced clear evidence that moving to a less socioeconomically disadvantaged area could benefit health, most notably by lowering obesity and diabetes.[30]

Specifically, compared to the control group that remained in public housing, people receiving both the traditional voucher and the voucher requiring and assisting in relocation to a low-poverty neighborhood showed sizable and significant proportional reductions of 15 to 20 percent in both morbid (BMI of 35 or higher) and very morbid (BMI of 40 or higher) obesity. People in the low-poverty voucher group (though not the traditional voucher group) also showed about a 20 percent reduction in diabetic levels of blood sugar (glycated hemoglobin of 6.5 or higher).

In sum, increasing evidence shows that the social context in which people live can significantly affect their health, though the evidence is not yet as extensive or strong across study populations or health outcomes as the evidence for the other policy areas considered in this chapter. And some impacts of the MTO program have been adverse, especially for the mental health of boys. Given this evidentiary base, the high level of both public and private policy focus on communities seems to reflect some greater sense of political palatability and tractability in this policy area, relative to the more starkly socioeconomic policy areas considered earlier, where the evidence shows stronger health impacts across a broader range of population health outcomes. Further, it is not clear that changes in communities (or the relocation of individuals) can be sustained without accompanying improvement in individuals' socioeconomic positions and reductions in the social institutional forces tending to perpetuate racial segregation in housing. In the end, we need to move to health in all policies and comparably broad health impact assessment, while especially targeting policies that are likely to have the largest and most pervasive effects in improving health and hence reducing spending for health care and insurance.

Conclusion

Evidence increasingly indicates that almost all forms of public policy have health effects and thus should be considered in relation to, and even as part of, health policy. This is what proponents of health in all policies and health impact assessment are seeking to achieve. Many of the effects of the nonhealth policies considered in this chapter are as large or larger than the effects of evidence-based medical care, and arguably more cost-effective. Better understanding and evaluating the health impacts of a wide range of public policies will also modify our sense of the costs and benefits of all these policies—in some cases quite radically.

Yet public policy also remains all about making choices and setting priorities. With respect to the overall goal of resolving America's paradoxical crisis of health and health policy, education and income policy merit special attention. They are well-established policy areas, together rivaling health policy in their size as a percentage of GDP. For both, we now have an impressive body of research documenting their consequential impacts on health, including the impacts of specific existing or potential policy programs. These policies are closely linked with other areas of policy—such as macroeconomic, civil rights, and housing and neighborhood policy—where the evidence of health effects is increasing. And we have seen that an even wider range of policies—agricultural, commercial, transportation, and others—are implicated in some of our major societal health problems, such as smoking and obesity and their sequelae.

The linchpin of a new demand-side health policy is improving levels of population health via nonhealth policies to reduce the need and demand for health care and hence expenditures on health care and insurance. This chapter has shown that a wide range of such policies can fundamentally and consequentially affect health. The next chapter seeks to show the economic benefits of a healthier population, especially in reducing expenditures for health care and insurance.

Chapter 8

The Economic Value and Impact of a New Demand-Side Health Policy

PART I of this book indicated that population health and health disparities are determined by social, environmental, behavioral, and psychological factors more than by health care and insurance. Chapters 6 and 7 showed why we have been able to improve population health and reduce health disparities more effectively through socioeconomic and other nonhealth policies than by just providing more and better health care. Our spending on health care and insurance is outstripping all other nations, however, approaching 20 percent of our gross domestic product (GDP) and creating fiscal crises for all levels of government, private-sector organizations, and many individuals, families, and households. Will a demand-side approach improve our ability to manage and reverse our current crisis of spending on health care and insurance? Research has only recently begun to address this question, but as the evidence comes in, the answer increasingly seems to be "yes."

The Economic Implications of Population Health

Economists' interest in health has grown apace with the development of their field and the health care expenditure crisis. Initially, economists viewed health mainly as one element of human capital that contributes to economic productivity by making workers better able to work hard, long, and productively.[1] Indeed, some have argued that it was the dramatic improvements in health of the past several centuries, driven largely by improved agricultural productivity and hence nutrition (recall from chapter 3 the work of Thomas McKeown), that made possible the industrial revolution and the concomitant growth in the world economy and population. Prior to the eighteenth century, nutrition levels for most people were insufficient for sustained work activity. Humans largely lived at basic subsistence levels and died of hunger or disease when nutrition levels fell below even that. Thus, growth in both human populations and life expectancy was minimal.[2]

As the health of nations has improved, so has their wealth. (The reverse is also true, as seen in part I, especially chapter 3). It is difficult to establish a precise economic value of the impact of health on economic productivity. It varies depending on the health indicators, the types of work and economic activity, and the contexts that shape the connections between these factors. For example, physical health and development are more important in societies driven by physical labor, while cognitive and mental health matter more in societies, like our own, that are driven by information and intellectual work. How strong the link is, in either case, depends on how much socioeconomic and political systems allow or ensure that healthier individuals can work in contexts and ways that are maximally productive.

For present purposes, however, we do not need to place a specific economic value on this aspect of health as human capital. Economic growth does not necessarily lead to reduced health care expenditures and may in fact tend to increase such expenditures. It does, however, increase total economic output, which can provide resources and mechanisms for investment and debt reduction across a wide variety of areas, including health care. On balance, then, it is likely that economic growth will help alleviate the fiscal health care crisis, indirectly or directly. How and how much will depend on how we choose to invest or consume the fruits of increased economic growth.

The Economic Value of Healthy Human Life

The Declaration of Independence considered "Life" a fundamental and inalienable human right, along with "Liberty" and the "pursuit of Happiness." As economists have also come to be interested in health as an important aspect of human welfare—which is the ultimate product of and rationale for economic activity—it has become important to put a monetary value on health as well as measure it, so that health can be compared to and combined with other forms of economic output or utility. Using various methods, economists and others have tended to converge on a value of $100,000 to $300,000 for a person-year of (reasonably good-quality) human life. Although this estimated value includes some of the value of the economic output enabled by health, it is more an indicator of the value of life to people as a consumption good—specifically, an estimate of how much a person would be willing to pay for an additional year of (reasonably good-quality) life.[3]

Putting a value on a person-year of life provides another, more monetarily precise, way of estimating the economic impact of improving population health. For example, what would be the economic value of eliminating socioeconomic disparities in life expectancy? This value has been recently estimated for educational disparities in mortality in the U.S. population age twenty-five (the age by which most people have completed their education) and older. Using national age- and education-specific estimates of mortality, combined with a conservative estimated value of $100,000 for a year of (reasonably healthy) life, the economic value of raising the life expectancy of the non-college-educated to the life expectancy of the college-educated was estimated to be about $1 trillion, or 7.7 percent of GDP. A similar exercise in reducing educational disparities in the European Union yielded comparable values of €1 trillion, or 9.5 percent of GDP. Both the estimated value of a life used in this exercise and other assumptions were generally conservative, making these probably lower-bound estimates. For example, if we use higher estimates of $200,000 to $300,000 per healthy (or quality-adjusted) life-year, the U.S. estimate is two to three times higher. The European Union study also estimated that about one-seventh of the €1 trillion total stemmed from potential increases in human capital as reflected in earnings; the rest of the value was in "consumption goods," or the value people get from living a relatively healthy year of life.[4]

These estimates do not take account of what it would cost in terms of health or nonhealth policies and programs to achieve these increases. Further, they do not directly or necessarily translate into any reductions in health care and insurance expenditures. What we really need is evidence that a healthier population uses less health care and thus spends less on health care and insurance. This is exactly what recent research suggests.

Are the Healthy and Advantaged Less Likely to Use Health Care?

It is not self-evident that a healthier population or one with fewer social disparities in health is a population with lower levels of utilization and expenditures for health care and insurance. Indeed, our intuition might suggest exactly the opposite, for at least a couple of reasons. First, socioeconomically advantaged people simply can afford to spend more on everything, including health care and insurance. Second, to the extent that medical care and insurance contribute to better health, we might expect that spending more on them would be what makes people healthy. Indeed, this belief is widespread, and it undergirds our current supply-side health policy. Similarly, it is assumed that the way to reduce social disparities in health is to increase access to, and hence utilization of, better-quality health care and insurance across socioeconomic, racial-ethnic, and gender groups.

Yet we know that at the level of population health this seemingly logical and self-evident assumption does not hold. Chapters 1 to 3 showed that, across nations, spending on health care and insurance is unrelated to variations in levels of population health, and it is even negatively related if the United States is included. This finding implies that it may also be true within nations that healthier people, who tend to be of higher socioeconomic status and members of advantaged racial-ethnic groups, spend less on medical care and insurance, in spite of having greater access to it and ability to pay for it. Counterintuitive though this may seem, the evidence increasingly shows this to be the case.

Annual Expenditures

There has been relatively little direct effort to establish whether healthier or socially or economically advantaged people have higher or lower expenditures on health care and insurance. Far more research has been done on whether the disadvantaged, both socioeconomically and by race-ethnicity, have equitable levels of access to, utilization of, and spending on medical care or insurance. One by-product of this research, however, is a set of findings that in both the United States and the European nations the less healthy and the socioeconomically and racially-ethnically disadvantaged have annual medical care expenditures that are considerably greater than the expenditures of their advantaged counterparts.

For example, in the United States the Medical Expenditure Panel Survey (MEPS)—the gold standard for estimating individual medical care costs—found that on average in 2004 the 9 percent of the U.S. working-age (age twenty-one to sixty-one) population with disabilities had total annual medical expenditures per person of $10,508—4.46 times the $2,256 for people with no disabilities.[5] For out-of-pocket expenses (as opposed to those covered by public or private insurance), the expenditures of people with disabilities were 2.89 times greater than they were for the non-disabled ($1,458 versus $504). As a percentage of family income, medical expenditures for the disabled were over five times (10.6 percent) the percentage for the non-disabled (2.1 percent). Another study using MEPS data to look at the entire U.S. population found that the 18 percent of the population with disabilities accounted for almost 27 percent of all health expenditures, and for 38 percent and 69 percent of all Medicare and Medicaid expenditures, respectively.[6]

Research in Finland and across nine nations in the European Union also indicates that illness is the major driver of individuals' levels of health care expenditures.[7] We know that disadvantaged socioeconomic and racial-ethnic groups are sicker than their more-advantaged counterparts and hence are also likely to utilize more, and often more expensive, medical care. For example, care is more expensive in emergency rooms, and those who utilize emergency rooms are more likely to be in poorer health (by a factor of 2:1) and to be socioeconomically or racial-ethnically disadvantaged (by a factor of about 1.5:1).[8]

Lifetime Expenditures

All the research just noted has been based on annual expenditures. Because health care expenditures are heavily concentrated toward the end of life, particularly the last year, what is true for average annual expenditures may not be true for lifetime health expenditures. Recent research on the effects of obesity (arguably a form of morbidity at its medium and higher levels, and certainly associated with significant morbidity, such as hypertension and diabetes) suggests that the sick (here the obese) have greater lifetime as well as annual health expenditures. Data on obesity at age fifty and older from the nationally representative Health and Retirement Survey (HRS) and a U.S. population projection model, based on the observed associations in HRS of obesity with sociodemographic factors, health, and health care spending, yield the results in figure 8.1. That figure shows how much more an obese person at each age will generate in total health care and Medicare costs over his or her life course compared to a non-obese person: people obese at age fifty are expected to have $15,000 more in lifetime health expenditures, people obese at age sixty

Figure 8.1 The Marginal Effect of Becoming Obese at Baseline on Lifetime Health Care and Medicare Costs

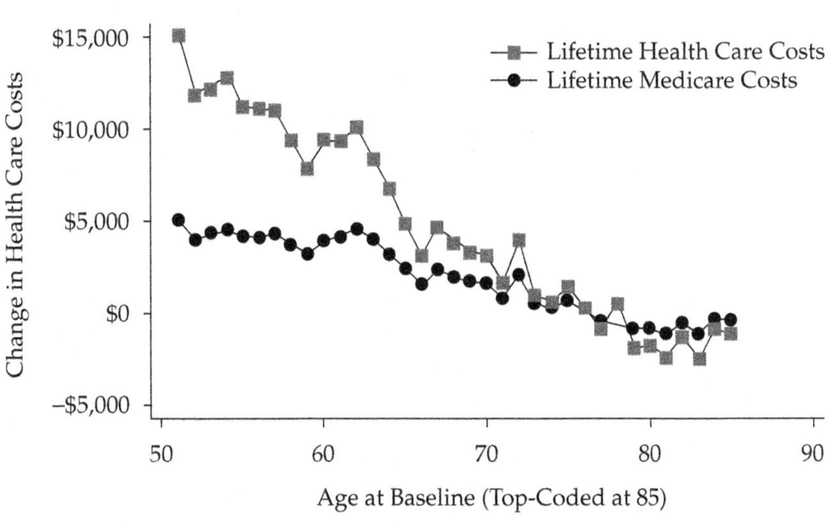

Source: Bhattacharya and Sood (2011, figure 4).

about $10,000 more, and people obese at age sixty-five about $5,000 more, with an excess cost of obesity no longer evident after about age seventy-five.[9] At age sixty-five, when the excess lifetime cost of obesity is about $5,000, Medicare begins to account for the vast bulk of all health care expenditures. However, Medicare spending accounts for only about one-third of the total excess lifetime health care costs for a person who is obese at age fifty.

The High Cost of Even a Small Health Problem

In 2009 I saw for myself how health care expenditures are driven by health problems that bring you into contact with the medical care system, especially its technology-intensive components. I have been fortunate to be a relatively healthy person most of my life, hospitalized only three times for common and routine surgeries—a hernia surgery and a tonsillectomy as a child and an appendectomy as a late adolescent. Costs for these kinds of routine medical procedures are relatively easily controlled by public and private insurance systems. Much more difficult to control are the costs for entries into the medical care system that involve long-term chronic care or more complex and uncertain diagnosis of potentially serious illness, both of which often require repeated visits and tests involving multiple specialists.

On a trip to India in 2009, I developed pneumonia (though probably from exposure before leaving), which first seemed like a common tourist's intestinal problem. When those symptoms disappeared and primarily respiratory ones remained, sinusitis was diagnosed, partly as a function of my own suggestion, based on sinusitis being the only serious respiratory illness I had ever had. After several weeks I was finally able to see my primary care physician, who diagnosed "walking" pneumonia, confirmed by chest X-ray, and sent me to the emergency room for evaluation and possible hospital admission. After five hours, I was released with antibiotics that cured the pneumonia. The cost of the ER visit: $2,000.

This was not, however, the end of my encounter with the medical care system. The chest X-ray revealed a possible small aortic enlargement that led to a $7,500 CT scan. Although it is not clear that I have a serious or progressive aortic problem, I am now receiving annual and biannual follow-up CT, MRI, and ultrasound scans at a cost of several thousand dollars per screening. And this was still not all. Although the CT scan indicated that the aortic problem was small, it also revealed spots on my lung. It turned out that these were the not-yet-resolved residue of my bout of pneumonia, not lung cancer. However, it took two visits to a pulmonologist and another chest CT scan to confirm this. By the end of this initial phase, my medical bills were approaching $20,000—the approximate total for almost all of my prior life. And I am now generating several thousand dollars of annual and biannual expenditures in order to monitor a *possibly* problematic aortic enlargement.

In sum, had I not had pneumonia, none of these expenditures would have occurred. Had it been correctly diagnosed and treated on my initial outpatient visit in India or the United States, the cost would probably have been $300 to $500. But once I entered the specialized and high-tech part of the medical care system, the cost of this illness quickly escalated into four and five figures, and it could get to six figures over my lifetime, even if the potential aortic problem never becomes clinically significant.

This was a first and only experience for me over a period of almost seven decades. For people whose conditions of life and work generate more actual or potential health problems that lead them into the specialized and high-tech part of the medical care system, this kind of experience occurs much more regularly. And these are people who are more likely to have no insurance or inadequate insurance and who thus have to pay more out of pocket. My own insurance works by first getting doctors and hospitals to accept less than the stated price, leaving me with little or no deductible to pay.

A Large-Scale Societal Projection

What might happen on a societal level if we were able to improve the overall health of the American population through changes in social life and policy outside the area of health care policy and practice?[10] A simple but compelling first approximation of this has recently been generated, using an enhanced version of a model developed at the RAND Corporation for simulating and predicting changes in the U.S. population age fifty and older (the same model that generated figure 8.1). Pierre-Carl Michaud, Dana Goldman, and their colleagues (2011) estimated the impact on both life expectancy and federal expenditures for Social Security, Medicare, and Medicaid if the health of the U.S. population age fifty and older gradually became equal over a period of thirty years to the average population health of eight other representative Organization for Economic Cooperation and Development nations—Denmark, France, Germany, Greece, Italy, the Netherlands, Spain, and Sweden—on self-reported measures of ten major morbidities and health risks: overweight, obesity, current and past smoking, heart disease, diabetes, stroke, lung cancer and other cancer, and hypertension.

This simulation of gradually improving the health of the American population increases life expectancy at age fifty by 1.2 years, essentially eliminating the current gap between Americans and Europeans age fifty and older. The model further indicates that virtually all of the increase is in healthy life expectancy rather than in prolonged survival in ill health, as one might expect if the cause of the increase in life expectancy was reduction in American rates of obesity, hypertension, diabetes, heart disease, cancer, and so on. This result also suggests that the health problems that are improved in this model well represent those health problems that affect mortality in later life. As noted again later, these problems may not encompass the full range of less life-threatening illnesses and disabilities that also contribute to our health and insurance expenditures.

The fiscal consequences for both federal and state government of such an improvement in healthy life expectancy among Americans age fifty and older are threefold. First, because healthier people live longer on average, they collect more Social Security benefits. Second, because they live longer and are healthier, they work more and for longer periods, thus generating increased tax revenues. Finally, because they are healthier, they use less medical care, which the federal and state governments pay for through Medicare and Medicaid. On a *lifetime* per capita basis, each American fifty-year-old is projected on average to pay $2,425 more in federal and state taxes, to receive $6,593 more in Social Security benefits, and to spend $17,791, or 8.5 percent, *less* on health care (of which $6,847, or about 30 percent, represents federal expenditures for Medicare, Medicaid, or disability insurance) than if his or her health level remained on its current trajectory.

Figure 8.2 shows how this all would unfold over time. Relative to the status quo, as America's population health came to approximate European health between 2004 and 2030, health expenditures would decline linearly and almost continuously, though at a diminishing rate after 2030 and especially after 2040, when the new fifty-year-old age cohorts would no longer be improving in health relative to their European counterparts (lower short and long dashed line). These savings in health expenditures would reach $60 billion or more *annually* in 2004 dollars by about the year 2040. Social Security costs would begin to increase after 2020 as the fifty-year-old cohorts with improving health since 2004 reached retirement age (middle dotted line). Even so, the change in total expenditures (the middle dashed line, which is simply the sum of the changes in spending for health and Social Security) would remain negative or zero until 2050, yielding a still-positive net fiscal saving (top solid line).

Figure 8.3 shows the cumulative effects of all this for the period between 2004 and 2050. The first two bars of figure 8.3 show that even as far out as 2050 the increased tax revenues from a healthier and longer-lived population would essentially pay for their increased Social Security benefits. The last two bars show that as of 2050 there would remain savings of $632 billion (2004 dollars) in Medicare ($328.29 billion) and Medicaid ($303.92 billion) expenditures, or about 1.6 years' worth of their current cost. Finally, the middle bars show additional savings by 2050 of almost $77 billion in disability benefits ($64.85 billion) and Social Security In-

Figure 8.2 The Thirty-Year Impact on Government Spending of Improving the Health for U.S. Adults Age Fifty and Older in 2006 to the Average Level of Comparable European Nations

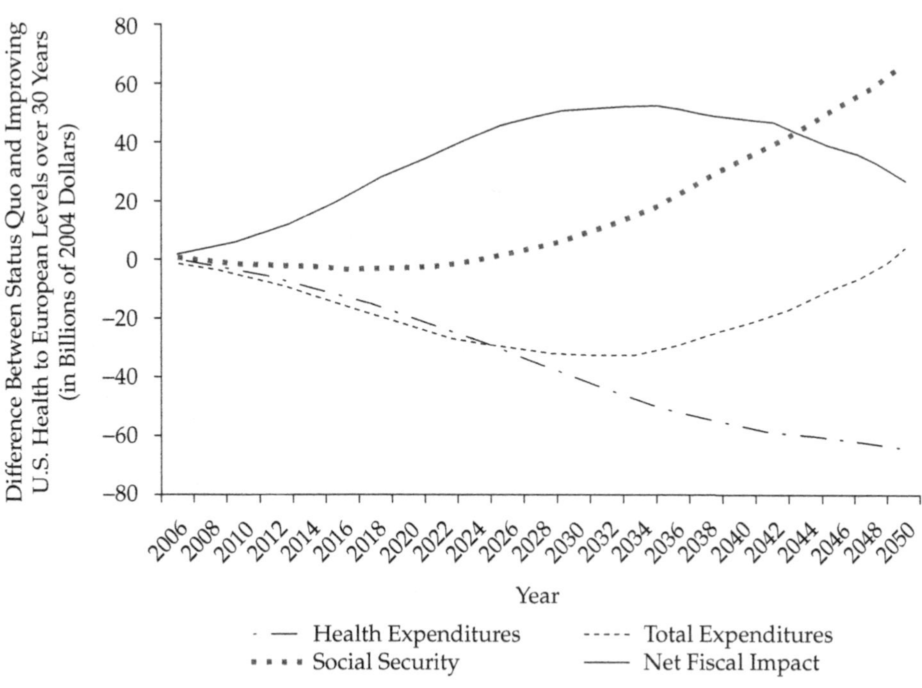

Source: Michaud et al. (2011, figure 5). © 2011 Elsevier Limited. Reprinted with permission.
Notes: Health expenditures include Medicare and Medicaid. Social Security includes SSI and OASDI expenditures. Net fiscal impact is the revenue change minus the total expenditure change. Calculated using the microsimulation model.

come (SSI) benefits for disabled elderly ($12.06 billion). This all implies over $1 trillion in savings from currently projected total health expenditures, both public and private.

These estimates are likely to be conservative, for several reasons. First, they deal only with the population over age fifty. Although the majority of medical care expenditures occur in the last twenty to thirty years of life, there are still significant health issues under age fifty, such as accidents, congenital disorders in children, or pregnancy care, that are not reflected in figures 8.1 and 8.2. Second, health improvement grinds to a complete halt in 2030 under this scenario, and subsequently improvements in population health and reductions in health care expenditures become muted. It is more likely, however, that the forces generating health improvement would continue and perhaps even strengthen after

Figure 8.3 The Effect of Bringing the Health of Americans Up to the Average Health of Comparable European Nations on the Present Discounted Value of Government Expenditures and Revenue, 2004–2050

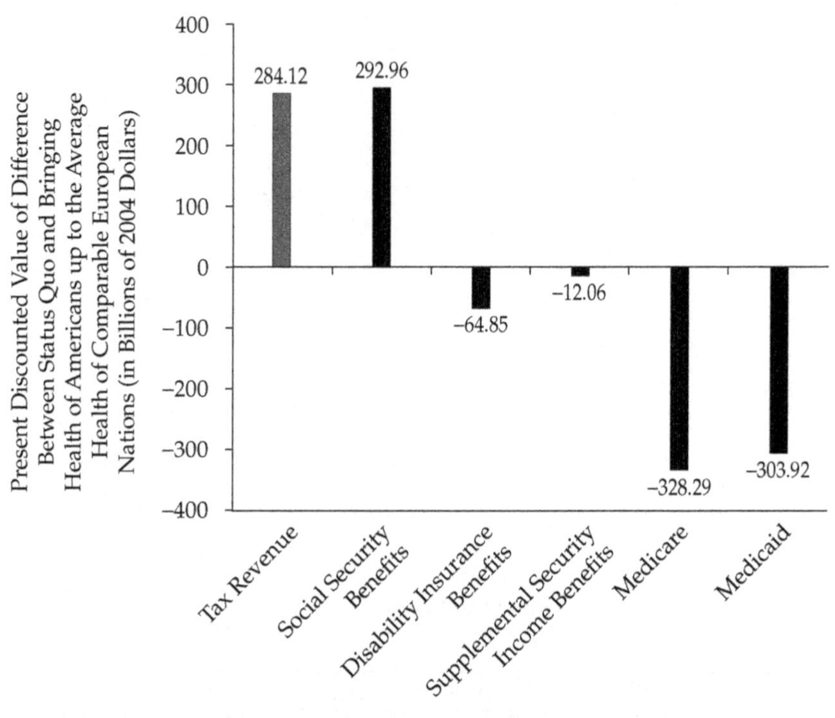

Source: Michaud et al. (2011, figure 6).
Notes: Present discounted value calculated using a 3 percent real discount rate from 2004 to 2050. Tax revenue includes federal, state, and Social Security and Medicare taxes. Calculated using the microsimulation model.

2030. Third, the model improves health on only ten health risk or disease indicators—albeit a major ten—and leaves out a whole range of other factors that would affect health spending (such as cognitive or musculoskeletal problems).

Does Better Health Reduce Health Care Spending?

In sum, studies of annual health care expenditures and projections of lifetime trajectories of health care spending as a function of different levels of health at age fifty both indicate that a healthy population generates a substantially lower level of health care spending. The projection models in figures 8.1 to 8.3—especially if extended to more diseases and risk factors, to persons under age fifty, and beyond 2030—would reduce total health care expenditures at least by 10 to 20 percent compared to models that assume the continuation of current trends in health and health risk factors. The studies that show greater spending among the less healthy and the disadvantaged suggest that spending reductions could be even greater if the social and health disparities of these groups were markedly reduced, even if not eliminated. Given the preliminary and conservative nature of the estimates presented here, the declines in expenditures associated with improving health more fully and more broadly are likely to rival, and ultimately exceed, even the most optimistic projected reductions in health expenditures under the current health care reform or proposed alternatives to or extensions of it.[11]

There are, of course, costs associated with improving health, even improvements driven by social and economic factors and policies. However, such policies—for example, education policy or transportation policy to reduce accidents—are likely to improve human capital, productivity, and other aspects of well-being, making these policies even more cost-effective. Given the uncertain magnitudes of the cost savings, if any, that are likely to accrue under the Affordable Care Act or proposed alternatives to it, a demand-side policy of improving population health via largely nonhealth policies offers our best chance of both improving population health and also substantially reducing the rate of growth in health spending, perhaps even to levels that would make the United States no longer an egregious outlier on either dimension among highly developed and wealthy nations.

We cannot abandon our efforts to achieve a more cost-effective health care and insurance system on the supply side—nor should we—but the initial estimates of the impact on health care expenditures of a demand-side policy to improve population health, largely through means other than health care, look even more promising. Moreover, reductions in expenditures from demand-side policy are associated with, and a function of, gains in health, whereas a supply-side approach only hopes that reducing medical care and insurance spending will not adversely affect health, and perhaps will improve health.

Further, recent evidence suggests that "nonclinical environmental" interventions aimed at preventing disease and ensuing disability or death are more cost-effective than "clinical and/or person-oriented interventions." Nonclinical environmental interventions are the kind of changes in broad public policy reviewed in chapter 7. They are interventions directed at large populations to promote health or prevent disease, rather than interventions delivered to individuals or in clinical settings (including disease and risk screening and even vaccination). A review and analysis of 2,815 cost-benefit analyses of preventive interventions published through 2011 compared their costs with the imputed dollar value of the increased quality-adjusted life-years they produced. Forty-six percent of environmental interventions cost less than the dollar value of their health benefit, while only 16 percent of clinical interventions and 13 percent of person-delivered nonclinical interventions were similarly cost-saving. Even for interventions that cost more than the dollar value of their health benefit, environmental interventions had better cost-benefit ratios. And whereas between 5 and 10 percent of clinical and person-centered nonclinical interventions were iatrogenic (they actually worsened health), none of the environmental interventions were.[12]

This study further indicates that the demand-side approach to health policy developed in chapters 6 and 7 has substantial positive outcomes in not only improving population health but also reducing the level of expenditures for health care and insurance, arguably to a greater degree and with more certainty than even the most optimistic scenarios for health care reforms focused on the supply side.

Chapter 9

Understanding and Resolving America's Paradoxical Crisis of Health Care and Health

POLITICAL STRUGGLES over Obamacare and the challenges in implementing it continue to preoccupy health policy in our nation. Yet, as seen in chapter 1, we face a more fundamental crisis in health policy, and in public policy more generally. We are spending more every year on health care and insurance, both absolutely and relative to all other nations, at levels that are increasingly burdening, and sometimes bankrupting, households, private organizations, and all levels of government. Yet the health of our population is declining relative to all comparably wealthy nations, and some less wealthy ones as well, and recently has even begun to decline absolutely for some portions of our population, such as lower-educated and -income women. We need a health policy that can simultaneously and effectively address both aspects of this paradoxical crisis.

Yet, as shown in chapter 2, Obamacare, or any attempt to reform health policy from the supply side by increasing access to health insurance and care while attempting to make these more cost-effective, will at best only marginally improve population health or control our burgeoning spending on health care. Disease and injury are prototypical of the kinds of unpredictable problems that should be dealt with by insurance, which should be as universal as possible, not only as a matter of social justice but in order to be as inexpensive as possible for each insured person and as economically feasible and cost-effective as possible for insurers. Thus, there is every reason to broaden health insurance coverage as much as possible and to make the almost 20 percent of our economy devoted to health care and insurance as cost-effective as possible. But we should also try to reduce the levels of insurable risks as much as possible, and that is why we need to promote population health. We should stop deluding ourselves that any reform of health care and insurance policy can at this point do much to alter either of the two central components of our paradoxical health policy crisis: burgeoning health spending and worsening population health outcomes.

The reasons for revising our approach are both tactical and strategic. Tactically, all past and current evidence and all sound and empirically based future projections indicate that efforts to broaden access to health care and insurance and make them more cost-effective face continuing and increasingly strong opposition from some political parties and factions and from an ever-growing medical-biotechnology complex. The history and current state of Obamacare make this abundantly clear. Yet there is a more fundamental and strategic flaw in a solely supply-side health policy, or any reform of it: the implicit, if not explicit, assumption of such policies and reforms that health care is the major determinant of population health. It is *not*. This assumption precludes any understanding that the major determinants of health reside in broader social factors and policy.

Chapter 3 indicated why we cling so tenaciously to the belief that health care is the major, even exclusive, determinant of population health. It also showed how and why the full range of scientific evidence suggests that health care probably never has accounted for more than 10 to 20 percent of the variance in population health, and especially changes in population health, at least in economically developed societies like the United States. The major determinants of the remarkable improvement in population health of the currently developed societies of the world over the past 250 or so years have been socioenvironmental and psychobehavioral factors that will continue to drive changes in population health.[1] Hence, these social, economic, environmental, behavioral, and psychological factors must become the central focus of a new demand-side health policy that seeks to improve population health through largely non-biomedical means, with the goal of developing a healthier population that needs and utilizes less health care and thus spends less on health care and insurance.

As seen in chapters 4 and 5, experience of and exposure to a broad range of socioenvironmental and psychobehavioral determinants of health are centrally driven by the major sources of social stratification and inequality in our society and others: socioeconomic position (especially education and income), race-ethnicity, and gender, or combinations thereof. The result has been wide social disparities in health by socioeconomic level, race-ethnicity, and, in more complex ways, gender, or combinations of all three. Whereas the most-advantaged portions of our population are approaching biologically maximal levels of health and longevity, the socially disadvantaged lag far behind and present the greatest opportunities for improving population health.

Education, income, and the socially constructed nature of race-ethnicity and gender are thus the primary levers for driving improvements in a very wide range of risk factors for health, and hence in overall population health. Social and health disparities by race-ethnicity and gender are often a function of associated socioeconomic deprivations. Thus, improving individuals' socioeconomic circumstances, especially their education and income, is a sine qua non for reducing all health disparities and improving population health—though factors unrelated to socioeconomic status that affect health and related racial-ethnic and gender disparities, such as discrimination and segregation, must also receive attention.

Chapters 6 and 7 reviewed the past and current research, both observational and experimental, that has demonstrated the ways in which a wide range of "nonhealth" policies have improved individual and population health, increasingly more cost-effectively than health care and insurance. The success of nonhealth policies in improving population health has led to calls for consideration of health in all policies (HiAP) and health impact assessments (HIAs) of all policies, though some policies, such as education and income, are more equal than others in this regard.

And as seen in chapter 8, an emerging body of research shows that better health leads to lower levels of spending on health care and insurance, at the level of both individuals and populations. Indeed, savings in health care and insurance expenditures in the trillions of dollars are projected to arise from simply bringing population health in the United States up to the average of comparable European countries, which can largely be done via broader socioeconomic policy. These levels of savings approximate the most optimistic goals of those seeking to reduce health care spending and overall government deficits. Thus, a demand-side health policy offers the promise of resolving our paradoxical crisis of health care and health and ending America's increasingly exceptional status relative to comparably wealthy nations in terms of both (growing) health care spending and (worsening) levels of population health. A demand-side health policy could also make major contributions to solving other social and fiscal problems in both the public and private sectors.

American Population Health in the Twentieth Century: Further Evidence for Addressing the Paradox with Demand-Side Policy

The review here of chapters 1 through 8 makes a strong case for developing a demand-side approach to health policy that will complement, but also come to rival or even exceed in scope, current supply-side approaches and reforms. Indeed, once we understand the argument presented in this book, we see that the history of America over the twentieth century arguably demonstrates that it is socioeconomic factors and policies that both brought our nation to a good and enviable place in terms of population health and spending on health by the third quarter of that century and have since driven us into the paradoxical crisis of health care and health that now threatens the health and economic well-being of our nation. Thus, these same socioeconomic factors and policies are the essential keys to resolving the crisis. Conclusively proving this proposition would take another book, but here we can make an argument, entirely consistent with the evidence presented in this book, for an increased focus on a demand-side health policy grounded in our understanding of the social determinants of and disparities in health.

America's Late-Twentieth-Century Shift in Health Spending, Population Health, and Socioeconomic Attainment

Even in the face of two world wars and the Great Depression, the first seven decades of the twentieth century were characterized by great improvements in the socioeconomic level and health of the American population, both absolutely and relative to other nations. National expenditures on health also grew, but not in ways that were particularly distinctive relative to other comparably wealthy nations. The 1970s and especially the early 1980s constituted a watershed moment when population health and the socioeconomic levels of many Americans stagnated noticeably relative to both other comparably developed nations and most prior decades of the twentieth century in America. At the same time, America's health spending took a markedly upward trajectory, both absolutely and relative to other developed nations. This can be seen for both health spending and population health in figures 1.1 to 1.8 of chapter 1.

Figure 1.1 shows that U.S. spending on health as a percentage of gross domestic product (GDP) was rising more or less in parallel with other nations up through 1970. But in the 1970s the United States began to outdistance all other nations in both percentage of GDP and per capita spending on health, and this trend only accelerated in the 1980s. Canada, in contrast, transitioned from parity with the United States to parity with other nations, perhaps as a result of instituting an essentially single-payer national health insurance system with associated controls on medical utilization and costs, something that is much harder to accomplish in the contemporary United States. Perhaps Canada also followed more health-promoting social policies of all types.

The rate of improvement in life expectancy for American males (figures 1.2 and 1.4) slowed after 1980, relative to the post-1980s trends for other nations. For American women (figures 1.3 and 1.5), the rate of increase in life expectancy slowed dramatically after 1980, relative to both the prior U.S. trajectory and the post-1980 trajectories of other nations. U.S. rates of infant mortality worsened markedly relative to other nations up to the early 1970s, improved absolutely and relatively during the 1970s (perhaps especially because of improvements in living and working conditions and health care for the black population), but then steadily worsened again relative to other nations after 1980 (figure 1.7). Maternal mortality also improved absolutely, if not relatively, into the 1970s, but then worsened both relative to other nations and also absolutely after 1980.

We know that spending on health care and insurance has some positive effects on health, albeit much less than commonly presumed, though the cost-effectiveness of this kind of spending has been declining over the past half-century or so. Thus, the worsening health trends of the last several decades are even more perplexing in relation to the burgeoning health spending. What can explain these seemingly paradoxical trends since the 1970s?

The analysis in chapters 1 to 8 would lead us to take a look at the changes in nonhealth policies, especially socioeconomic ones, that began in the 1970s and accelerated thereafter. Many previously regulated aspects of the economy, including health care but also airlines, telephone service, and ultimately financial institutions, were deregulated over time. In a number of cases, the result was decreasing prices and increased consumption. In health care and insurance, however, consumption grew without a decrease in prices, reflecting the increased utilization of more expensive technology in health care. This trend, which continues to this day, can be significantly stemmed only by making the population healthier and thus less likely to need care in the high-technology arenas of our health care and insurance system.

The End of Rising Levels of Secondary and Postsecondary Education

More importantly, marked deteriorations in some key social determinants of health became apparent by the 1970s; the deterioration was reinforced in the 1980s and has not yet really been reversed. Most notable were changes in the two determinants we have identified as probably most important for health—education and income. Figures 9.1 and 9.2 show high school and college graduation rates, respectively, by cohorts of Americans who had had their twenty-first birthday at the beginning of each decade of the twentieth century, as well as various sociodemographic subgroups within each cohort. As we have seen, high school and college graduation are particularly consequential for health and its risk factors.

The improvements in these outcomes over the first seventy or so years of the twentieth century were dramatic, as was the almost complete stag-

Figure 9.1 High School Graduation Rates for All and by Gender, Region, and Racial Ancestry, by Year of Twenty-First Birthday, United States, 1900–2000

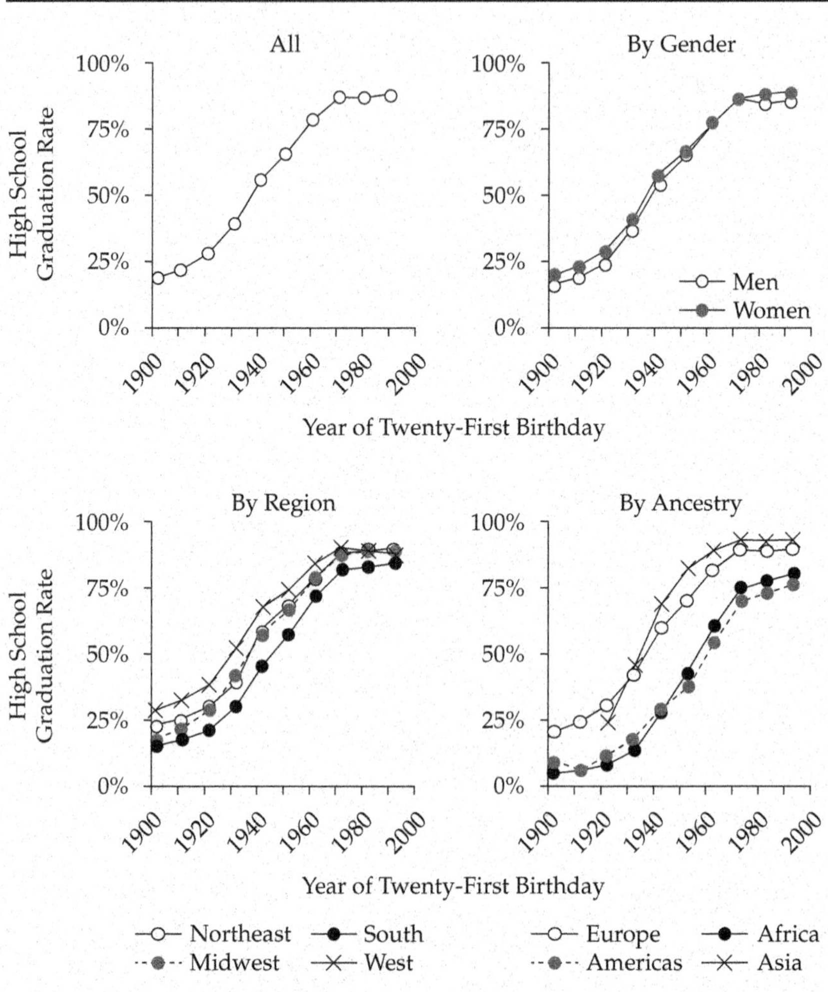

Source: Fischer and Hout (2006, figure 2.2), from Integrated Public Use Microdata Series (IPUMS) data.

Notes: The data for the 1900 and 1910 cohorts contain too few Asian Americans to yield a reliable estimate.

Figure 9.2 College Graduation Rates for All and by Gender, Region, and Ancestry, by Year of Twenty-First Birthday, United States, 1900–2000

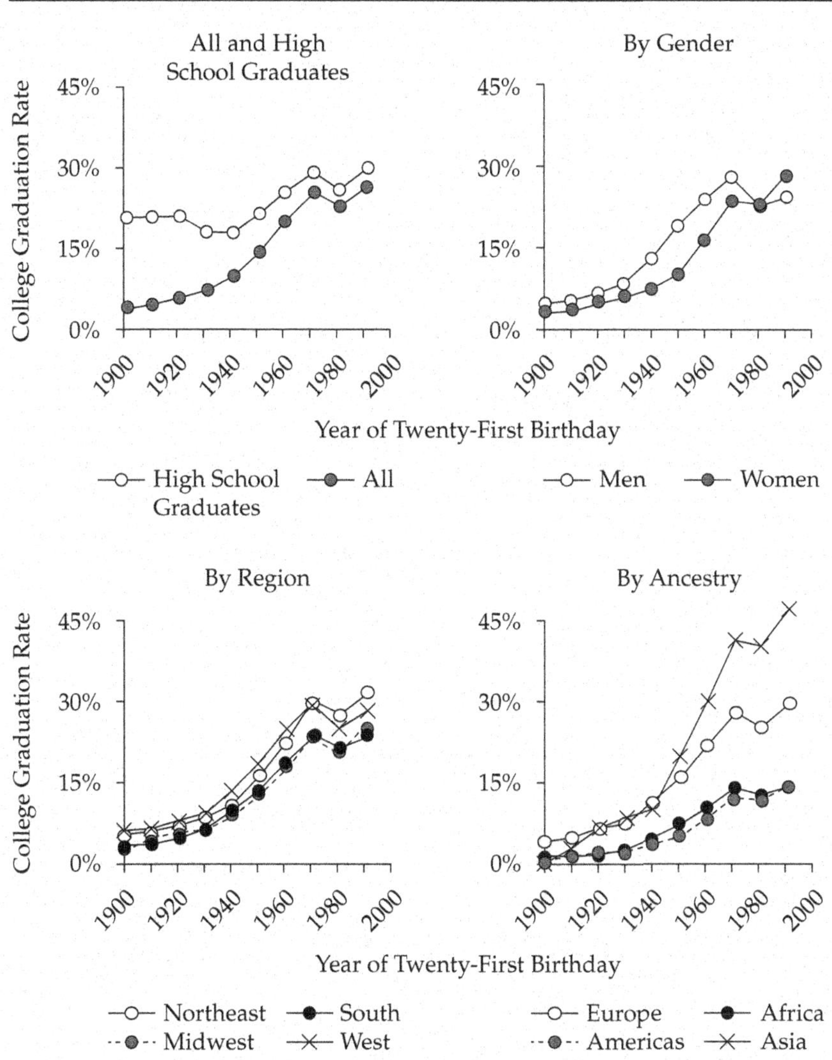

Source: Fischer and Hout (2006, figure 2.3), from IPUMS data.
Notes: The data for the 1900 and 1910 cohorts contain too few Asian Americans to yield a reliable estimate.

nation in these gains beginning with the 1970 cohort. Subject to some fluctuation with the economy, this growth followed by stagnation characterizes all of the segments of the U.S. population considered in figures 9.1 and 9.2, with the notable exception of college graduation for Asian Americans, which suffered only a brief hiatus in growth between 1970 and 1980. Also worth noting, in the upper left quadrant of figure 9.2, is that most of the gains in college graduation were made largely after 1940, presumably after World War II, reflecting a sharp rise in the proportion of high school graduates going to college via the GI Bill and subsequent federal aid mechanisms, in conjunction with a vast expansion of public higher education at the state level.

The reasons for this relatively abrupt cessation in the 1970s of the growth of education in the American population (with associated declines in quality, as discussed in chapter 7) are complex and not fully understood. Very important, however, must be the declining rates of increase in public funding of primary, secondary, and especially postsecondary education at the state and local levels; these declines were not sufficiently compensated for by the continuing growth of funding support at the federal level.[2] At the college level, there was also a major shift away from parental, institutional, and government payment-as-you-go for higher education to a system of financing dependent on loans to students. The result is a population in which education levels have not been growing since 1970 and whose debt levels are rising, compounding our paradoxical crisis in health policy and broader problems of public policy. Over the past two decades, we have seen levels of education for women growing once again.

In sum, dramatic increases in rates of graduation from high school (from about 20 percent in 1900 to 80 percent by 1970) and college (from less than 5 percent in 1900 to almost 30 percent by 1970) undoubtedly were major stimuli to the dramatic improvements in the health of the American population over the first seventy-five years of the twentieth century. And the almost complete cessation of such educational gains after 1970 is undoubtedly a major factor in the deterioration of the rates of gain in health since then—and hence the increasing need and expenditures for health care and insurance.

The United States led the world for most of the twentieth century in rates of both high school and college graduation. Today we have fallen to about the middle of the Organization for Economic Cooperation and Development (OECD) nations on such indicators, reflecting the deterioration in educational opportunity and attainment for the cohorts born since 1950 that is evident in figures 9.1 and 9.2. How far we have declined in this regard relative to other nations has been strikingly captured in a recent OECD report using data that are eerily similar to America's levels of population health relative to other nations. Figure 9.3 shows twenty-four

Figure 9.3 Educational Mobility Among Nonstudents Age Twenty-Five to Sixty-Four, by Country, 2012

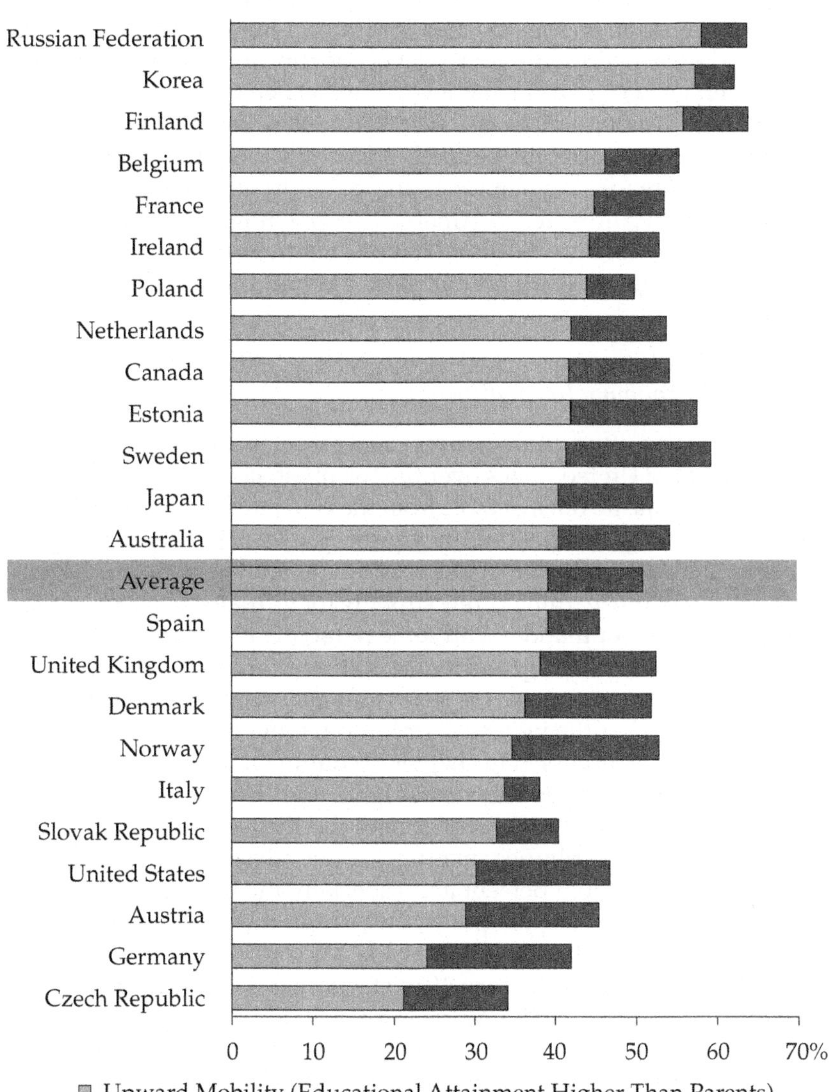

Source: OECD (2014, chart A.4.3).
Note: Countries are ranked in descending order of proportion of adults with upward mobility with respect to the educational attainment of their parents.

OECD nations ordered by the percentages in 2012 of twenty-five- to sixty-four-year-old adults not still in school whose educational attainment was higher than their parents. The United States ranks twenty-first out of twenty-four nations on this indicator. Only 30 percent of U.S. adults had exceeded their parents' levels of education, compared to an OECD average of 40 percent and levels over 50 percent in Russia, Korea, and Finland. Although more research is needed to establish clear causal connections, it is entirely reasonable that the worsening of education levels across America's generations compared to other comparable nations is a significant factor in America's worsening population health relative to other nations, recalling that our relative standing on population health indicators is highest at older ages and declines at younger ages.

Income and Economic Inequality

A very similar picture characterizes changes in income and economic inequality in the United States over the twentieth century. Good income and earnings data are not available from the U.S. census prior to 1940, but we can reasonably assume that they grew between 1900 and 1930 and probably fell during the Great Depression. As shown in figure 9.4, between 1940 and 1970 earnings grew strongly for virtually all major groups of workers in the population, with some reduction in inequality—that is, the distance between the top and bottom fifths of the income distribution. But earnings, like education, essentially stagnated after 1970, except at the very high end of the income distribution, though women (and African Americans, as discussed in chapter 7) continued to make some progress owing to advances in their civil rights and hence their labor force opportunities. Inequality in earnings between the top and bottom quintiles of the income distribution increased, especially among men and full-time workers. The top 5 percent and especially the top 1 percent of the population have dramatically pulled away from those below in terms of both income and wealth.[3]

A full explanation of the post-1980 stagnation of earnings is beyond the scope of this book, but a few historical trends can be noted. One has been a shift in the structure of the economy away from manufacturing and toward service, finance, and high-technology industries and jobs. This shift has made education even more central to economic success. At the same time, the key factors that had previously increased and sustained the earnings of less-educated workers have eroded, especially the minimum wage (beginning in the 1970s and accelerating after 1980, as shown in figure 9.5) and the size and influence of labor unions. Union membership declined from about one-third of the labor force in the 1950s to 25 percent in 1980 to less than 10 percent today.[4]

Figure 9.4 Earnings at the Twentieth Percentile, the Median, and the Eightieth Percentile, by Year and Gender, United States, 1940–2000

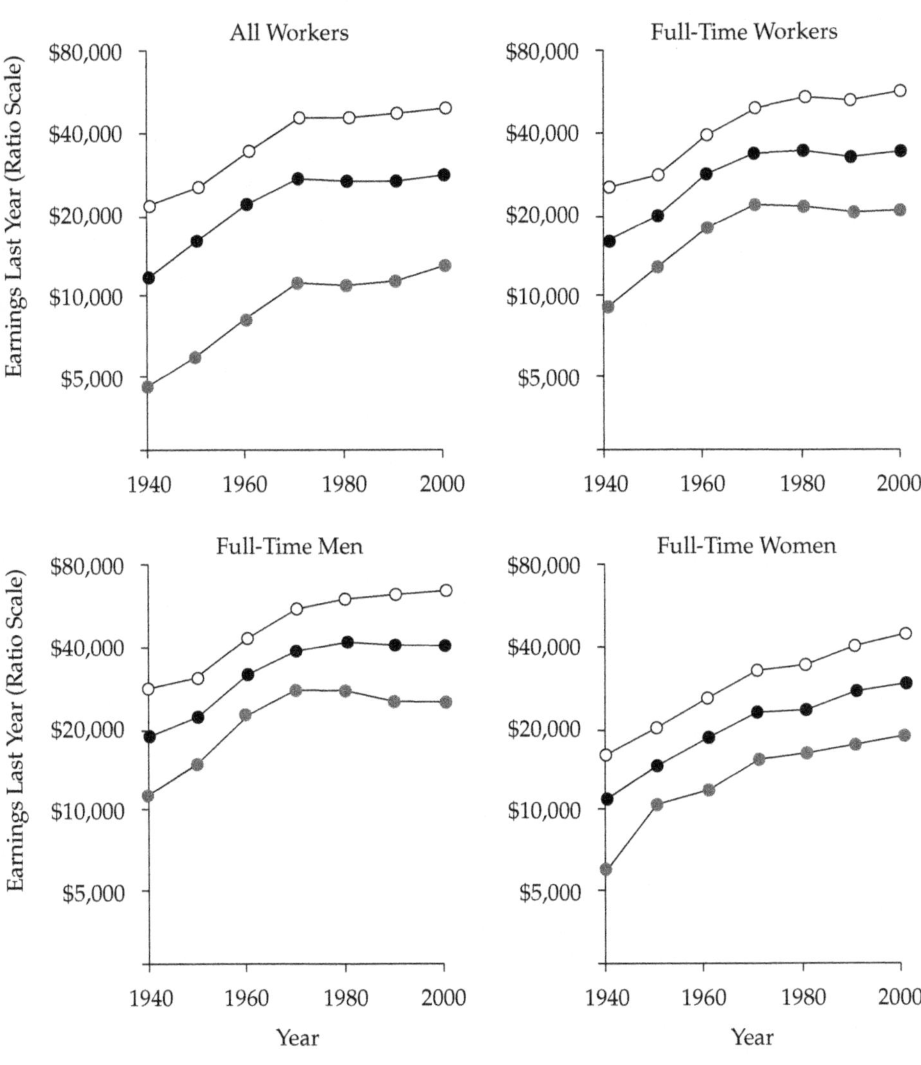

Source: Fischer and Hout (2006, figure 5.10), from IPUMS data.

Again, the strong growth in earnings over the first three-quarters of the century arguably had similar implications for health and health spending as the growth in education. The stagnation of earnings (in real dollars) as well as education that began in the 1970s have quite likely contributed importantly to the adverse trends in population health and

Figure 9.5 Real Purchasing Power of the Minimum Wage, United States, 1930–2000

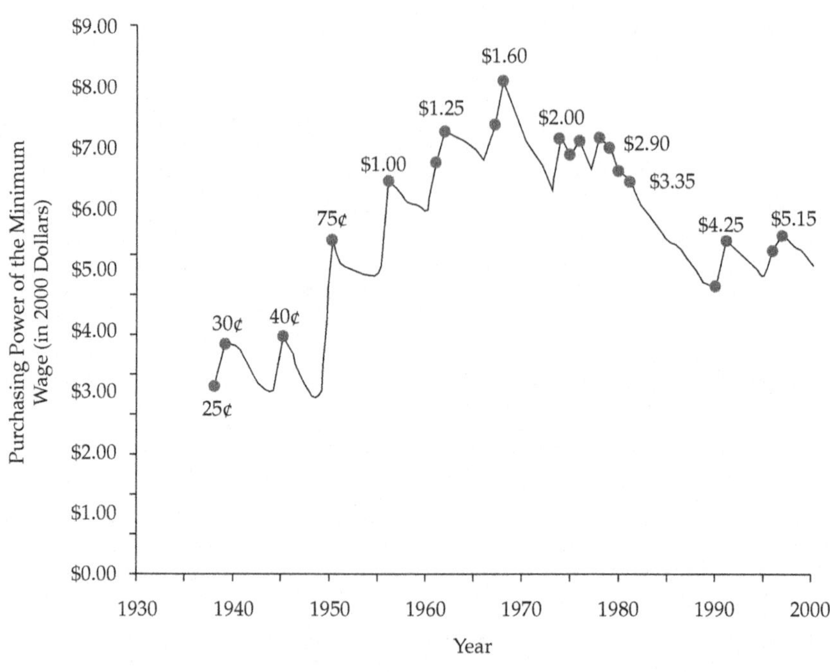

Source: Fischer and Hout (2006, figure 5.11), from IPUMS data.
Note: Dots show when the minimum wage was changed; labels show the nominal minimum wage in the year it first took effect.

health spending since 1980. Tax policy—from decreases in the progressivity of taxes to the taxation of earnings at a higher rate than capital gains—reinforced these other trends.

Family incomes continued to rise, though more slowly after 1970 than before, and at greater rates for households in the top income quartile, again increasing economic inequality. Family income growth was better than the growth of earnings only because so many women were entering the labor force. Their labor force participation produced a sharp increase in total hours worked in two-person/married households after 1975, even households with children, as seen in figure 9.6. That two people in the household have essentially been doing three jobs (two in the paid labor force and one unpaid job in the household) since 1975 rather than the two jobs that were previously typical (one in the labor force, one in the household) may also be a factor contributing to the deterioration of gains in life expectancy, especially for women, since 1980.

In sum, rising levels of education and income undoubtedly played a

Figure 9.6 Hours at Paid Work (Husband and Wife Combined) for U.S. Married Persons, Age Twenty-Five to Fifty-Four, Living in a Married-Couple Household, by Presence of Children in the Household, 1965–2000

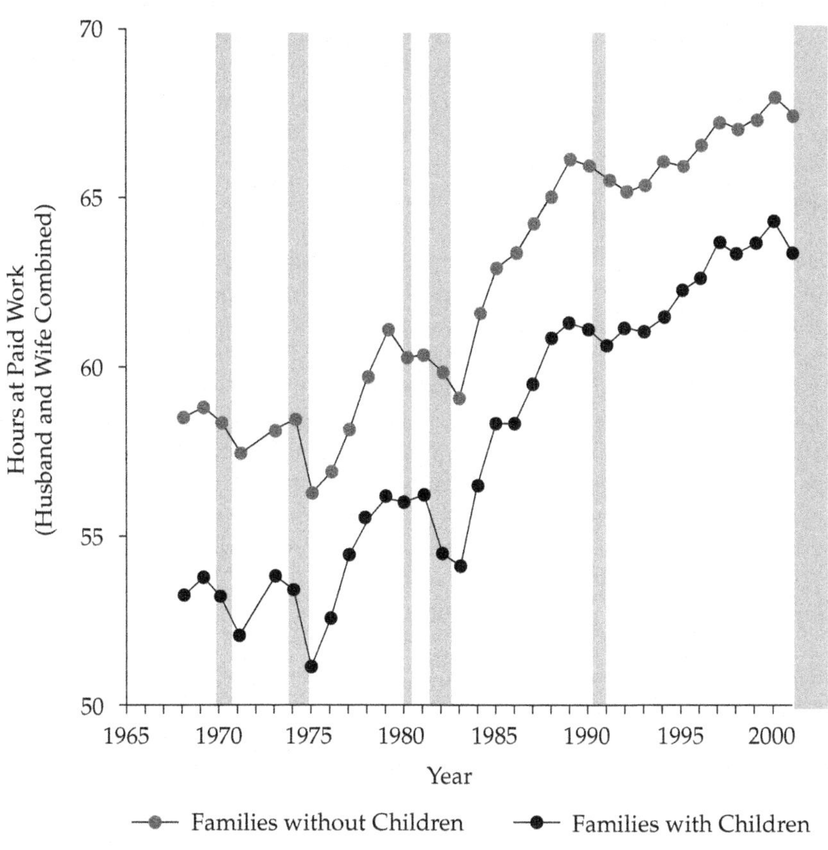

Source: Fischer and Hout (2006, figure 5.13), from Current Population Survey data.
Note: Gray stripes indicate recessions.

major role in the dramatic improvements in health and life expectancy over the first seven to eight decades of the twentieth century, probably much more so than the still-consequential improvements in the quantity and quality of health care and insurance over that period, as discussed in chapter 3. The rather abrupt halt of such increases, beginning in the 1970s and certainly since 1980, have arguably played a major role in the dramatic slowing of improvement in population health in America since 1980 and contributed to the dramatic increases in spending on health care and insurance.

This book makes the case that we can only resolve our paradoxical crisis of spending more and more on health care and insurance yet getting less and less in terms of population health via a new demand-side approach to health policy based on understanding social determinants and disparities of health and affirming their centrality to health policy. Our examination of public and private nonhealth policies before and since 1980 has strongly buttressed this case by suggesting that shifts in these very policies have helped to create the paradoxical crisis we now confront, just as they helped to create the more favorable trends in health and health spending in America prior to the 1970s.[5]

What Is to Be Done?

Chapters 1 to 6 showed that the only way to resolve America's paradoxical crisis of health care and health is to implement a strong demand-side health policy, using largely nonhealth policies to improve population health, which, as shown in chapter 8, can dramatically reduce levels of spending for health care and insurance. In contrast, as discussed in chapter 2, supply-side health policy and reforms, including the Affordable Care Act (ACA), that aim to make more and better health care and insurance available to more and more Americans, important as they are on a number of grounds, are unlikely to improve population health or reduce expenditures for health care and insurance more than marginally.

Cost-Effectively Targeted HIA and HiAP

Chapter 7 showed that a very wide range of public and private policies beyond health care and insurance can meaningfully improve population health. This conclusion is congruent with current movements toward health impact assessments, which evaluate the health impact of all policies, and health in all policies, which considers health impacts in formulating, projecting, and assessing the costs and benefits of all policies. HIA and HiAP promise to markedly expand and improve not only health policy but also understanding and analysis of the cost-effectiveness of nonhealth policies.

The problem with the broad HIA and HiAP initiatives at this point is that they do not sufficiently prioritize or target the nonhealth policies that most merit assessment of their health impacts and consideration of these impacts in formulating future policy. The analysis in chapter 7, reinforced by the data in figures 9.1 to 9.6 and the theory and evidence presented in chapters 4 and 5, clearly leads toward such a prioritization of socioeconomic policies related to education and income, as well as to civil rights and macroeconomic policy, though attention must certainly continue to be paid to a broader range of policies, including agriculture, environment, housing and urban development, and transportation.

HIA should be considered at least briefly in the implementation or change of any public policy, but actually pursued only in those cases where existing evidence suggests potentially significant health effects—for example, effects that at least approximate those required for approval of new drugs or medical procedures. Full-scale HiAP should be undertaken where the evidence from HIA and other research suggests potentially quite substantial impacts on health—of the magnitudes evident for well-established health behaviors (smoking, drinking, physical activity, and calorie consumption, weight, and obesity) and the policy areas considered in chapter 7. There is a growing need for research on such health impacts. This research could include joint ventures between major health agencies and major fiscal agencies at federal, state, and even local levels (and their private counterparts), for many of which expenditures on health are currently the single biggest source of fiscal problems.

From Research and Assessment to Policy: Strategic and Tactical Choices

While more research on the policy issues discussed in this book will always be needed, along with better and broader education regarding health, we have a pressing need—and enough understanding and evidence already—to begin to pursue policies that can help to resolve our paradoxical crisis of health and health care. These policies will also contribute more broadly to improving public and private policy regarding the most pressing social and economic problems of our time.

In thinking about the enactment and implementation of specific health and nonhealth policies, I continue to find very compelling John Kingdon's analyses of agenda-setting and policy formation, discussed in chapter 7 with respect to health care reform. Recall that Kingdon sees significant change in public policy as resulting from the confluence at a given moment in time of three "streams": the problem stream, the policy stream, and the political stream. It is important to consider how one's own and others' work contributes to or influences each of these streams and to recognize that few are likely to play a significant role in all three.

As a health scientist, I see my work as a contribution to defining and understanding a major social and political problem of contemporary America, what I have termed our "paradoxical crisis of health care and health." As a policy analyst, I draw on scientific research and analysis, both my own and that of others, to formulate policy recommendations that can help to address defined social, political, and policy problems—here a demand-side approach to health policy and to specific priorities and aspects of it. Nothing consequential happens until a well-defined problem amenable to some well-defined set of policy solutions intersects with a political stream that makes it possible to address the problem via the proposed policy solutions. As a citizen or member of an organization or enterprise, I can participate in and influence that political stream. As a scientist and policy analyst, however, my influence on the political stream can and should only derive from the problem and policy definitions I contribute proving attractive and useful to the actors in the political stream.

Additionally, I believe that my analysis and understanding of a societal problem and potential policies that can ameliorate it should not be primarily or heavily driven by my estimate, or anyone else's, of when and to what degree the political stream will be amenable to embracing my problem definitions and solutions, though I do hope that my ideas and evidence will be attended to by that stream in their consideration of political action. Kingdon has argued compellingly that his model explains how, why, and when we got the kind of health care and insurance policy and health care reforms that we have. It is likely that his model also explains when, how, and why the political stream may turn toward demand-side health policy.[6]

Chapter 7 defined a set of ordered criteria for identifying and prioritizing areas of social and economic policy as key components of health policy. On these grounds, I have prioritized education policy (at all levels), income policy, civil rights policy, and socioeconomic policy, while also recognizing the utility of a number of other policy areas. Within each of these, chapter 7 identified a range of specific policies that have established evidence and track records of their substantial impact on population health and ability to reduce the need for and utilization of health care, with consequent reductions in expenditures for health care and insurance. It should be noted that most of these policies were developed with bipartisan support at the national, state, and local levels—for example, policies promoting public education at all levels; income support policies such as Social Security Income (SSI), the Earned Income Tax Credit (EITC), and food stamps; civil rights policy; and macroeconomic policy with a dual goal of promoting low inflation and full employment. Other policies can be developed for these same purposes, also with bipartisan sources and support. Any of these programs can be part of a demand-side health policy, and indeed, their maintenance, restoration, and even enhancement in light of the trends we have discussed in this chapter are essential to such a policy.[7]

As was true for the political process that resulted in the ACA, ultimately the political stream will draw on the policies identified by the policy stream as capable of addressing and resolving the problems discussed in this book. I believe that chapter 7 gives the political stream a good menu to draw upon in this way. My current favorites would include, on the income side, maintenance of Social Security and enhancement of EITC, SSI, and food stamps, and on the education side, continued federal support as well as restoration of the large reductions in state and local support for education *at all levels,* as well as enhancements of support for the care and education of preschool-age children. These policies could be financed at first through more progressive taxation and ultimately with the savings from reducing expenditures on health.

Too often, I am afraid, contemporary efforts to improve population health and reduce health disparities, both within and outside of government, have stood criteria spelled out in chapter 7 (p. 108) on their head: dismissing the actions and policies advocated here as politically unpalatable and unfeasible, regardless of the extent to which those actions and policies meet the other criteria, all of which I regard as more important.[8] Again drawing on Kingdon, I would argue that it is most important that scientists and policy analysts provide the most evidence-based problem definitions and policy formulations possible and try to make them relevant to a broad range of political actors without constraining policy analysis to accommodate whatever forces may be momentarily holding sway in the political stream. The dramatic shift in civil rights policy with respect to race-ethnicity, gender, age, and sexual orientation over the past half-century indicates how relatively quickly political pendulums can swing, as do changes in socioeconomic, health, and other policy areas. Growing concern about inequality, apart from the issue of health disparities highlighted in this book, is increasing the chances of such broad changes in the social policies that have fundamental impacts on health. The growing bottom-up movement for increases in the minimum wage also represents a quite recent shift toward such policies. My hope is that, for the good of American society, the shift toward demand-side health policy along the lines developed here will come sooner rather than later, and that this book will contribute toward that end.

Conclusion

In documenting the paradoxical crisis in American health policy—we spend more and more on health care and insurance but get less and less in terms of population health—this book has demonstrated that Obamacare, or any health policy reform focused exclusively on the supply side of health care and insurance, cannot significantly affect, much less resolve, either part of this paradoxical crisis. This book has also demonstrated that a demand-side policy of improving population health and reducing social disparities in health, largely through nonhealth (socioeconomic, environmental, psychosocial, and behavioral) policies, shows every indication of being able to significantly improve population health and hence reduce the need for health care and actual spending on health care and insurance.

The case for a demand-side approach is predicated on the recognition that broader social and economic factors and policies, not health care and insurance are the major determinants of population health. The next step is recognizing that the surest way to reduce the utilization of and expenditures for health care is to reduce the need and demand for that care by making our population healthier via social and economic policy.

This chapter has reinforced the book's argument that our paradoxical crisis has developed and worsened as much as it has since the 1970s very plausibly because of our nonhealth policies since then—particularly our failure to improve education and income for the vast majority of the population, as we did throughout the first three-quarters of the twentieth century. These policies have created a less healthy population that needs more care at the same time that the technological intensity and cost of such care have been rising.

Reversal of these nonhealth policies—especially a return to policies focused on gains in education and income for the broad range of the population, not just an elite few—could improve our population health, both absolutely and relative to other nations. Such a change of direction in our policymaking would then begin to truly resolve our paradoxical crisis of health care and health by reducing expenditures for health care and insurance.

Changes in nonhealth policies could also simultaneously facilitate other desirable outcomes: improving the education and human capital of our country, our conditions of life and work (and play in the case of children), and the quality and healthfulness of our communities. In conclusion, much as Rudolph Virchow suggested in 1848, we cannot have efficient and effective health policy without effective and efficient social policies, and vice versa.

Notes

Preface

1. Quoted in Cassel (1976), from Frost (1936). John Snow is famous for mitigating a cholera epidemic in London in 1854 by taking the handle off the pump of the contaminated well.

Chapter 1

1. In figures 1.1 to 1.5 and 1.7 to 1.8, the United States is compared with four purposively selected other nations: Switzerland is our closest rival in terms of spending on health. Canada is the nation arguably most similar to the United States geographically, politically, socially, and culturally. The United Kingdom and Japan are two relatively low spenders on health care, with the former having many similarities and affinities to the United States and the latter being quite different historically, geographically, ethnically, socially, and culturally, as well as manifesting a unique and remarkable pattern of improvement in population health over the past half-century.
2. One can observe for the United States and the other nations a flattening of the upward trend in the years 2010 through 2012. This is primarily due to the Great Recession of 2007–2008, and hence government projections assume a return toward pre-recession growth rates in the last half of the current decade. Some argue, however, that health care reform and other changes in the health insurance and care systems may also be factors in the slowing rate of growth, as further discussed in chapter 2. Either way, growth in expenditures in the United States appears already to be resuming, and probably at a higher rate than in any comparable nation. Thus, the basic trend of U.S. divergence from all other nations in terms of GDP spent on health will continue—though whether at the same or a lower (or higher) rate than seen in the prior several decades remains to be seen.
3. To my knowledge, "medical-biotechnology complex" is a neologism, as a Google search reveals no evidence of prior usage, much less widespread usage. The notion is related to Arnold Relman's (1980) idea of a "medical-industrial complex." The new term more clearly incorporates the burgeoning biotechnology industry along with Relman's focus on hospitals, health care systems, pharmaceutical and medical device companies, and, increas-

ingly, the medical profession itself. Right up until his recent death, Relman focused most heavily on the for-profit health sector, though he increasingly recognized that the nonprofit health sector is also market-driven and distorted by that (see Relman 1991, 2014). He saw the essential American health care paradox as high expenditures coupled with still-limited access and proposed that it could be resolved with a single-payer insurance system and a return to greater professional autonomy of the medical profession. In my formulation, the entire health care and insurance system—nonprofit and for-profit, governmental and even university-affiliated—is part of the medical-biotechnology complex, and the American paradox is not just health expenditures versus access, but expenditures versus population health. This paradox, I argue, is not resolvable on the supply side by even a single-payer system and the enlightened leadership of the medical profession, desirable as both might be.

4. As this book was being prepared, the National Research Council (NRC) of the National Academy of Sciences and the Institute of Medicine released two major reports documenting the declining level of American population health, especially among women, relative to all comparably wealthy nations and to some less wealthy ones as well (National Research Council 2011a, 2011c; National Research Council and Institute of Medicine 2013). These reports confirm that the decline is evident for men as well as women, and for the elderly as well as the younger portions of the American population. Just as the Great Recession reduced spending on health and in many other areas, it may also paradoxically have increased life expectancy, for reasons that are discussed in chapter 7. Briefly, life expectancy tends to increase in recessions and even depressions and to decline during economic expansion, because recession reduces a broad range of risk factors for health, while expansion increases these risk factors. Most notable and intuitive is a decrease in driving and hence also highway accidents and fatalities during economic downturns and an upturn in driving, with correspondingly more accidents and fatalities, during economic upturns.
5. This possibility is implied in the NRC reports (National Research Council 2011a, 2011c; National Research Council and Institute of Medicine 2013) and confirmed for more than 43 percent of American counties, predominantly in the South (Kindig and Cheng 2013); earlier, Sandeep Kulkarni and his colleagues (2011) saw the same decline in 20 percent of U.S. counties. Many of these counties are admittedly small, and hence not fully reliable indicators. However, mortality experience has worsened for most of the female population nationally, with clear absolute declines for low-educated white women, as shown in figure 1.6 (Montez et al. 2011; Olshansky et al. 2012).
6. As discussed in chapter 3 and elsewhere, preventive medical care and public health will continue to play significant roles in improving population health. But health care, public health, and broader health policy need to recognize and incorporate a vastly broader range of nonmedical determinants of health.
7. Since James Fries (1980) proposed thinking about population health and health change as a process of extending or "compressing" human mortality, morbidity, and disability toward a biologically determined and finite human

life span, there has been great controversy over the limits of human life span and life expectancy and the mutability of these limits (see, for example, *Gerontologica Perspecta* 1987). No claims are made here about the potential mutability of current apparent biological limits on human life span or about how close life expectancy can come to approaching the maximal human life span. What is claimed is: (1) that there is now and always will be some biological limit; (2) that improving human health involves extending life expectancy toward that limit (as well as increasing the number of active and healthy years of that life expectancy and decreasing the functionally limited years); and (3) that the degree to which life and health can be extended or compressed toward the biological limit varies within and among human populations, with the more advantaged tending to be much closer to the limit than the less advantaged. For a reasonable discussion of many of these issues, which will be considered further in chapter 4, see the Wikipedia entry on life expectancy at: http://en.wikipedia.org/wiki/Life_expectancy.

8. As will be discussed in chapter 4, people who are more advantaged in terms of socioeconomic position, race-ethnicity, or gender are not immune to health hazards. For example, cigarette smoking was initially taken up first and most by upper socioeconomic white males. However, at every point in recent history, experience of and exposure to health hazards have been much greater among the less-advantaged portions of our society. Thus, since the late 1960s, smoking has become more prevalent among the lower socioeconomic strata, women, and some minorities.
9. As will be discussed in chapters 2 and 3, considerable evidence suggests that medical care and insurance are less important determinants of overall levels of population health than is commonly assumed. However, insurance and the access to care it provides have measurable positive impacts on health, not only in terms of mortality and life expectancy but also in making life with illness more manageable and productive, especially for the sickest and least-advantaged members of the population.
10. Others have also begun to argue for changes in health policy to take greater account of social determinants and, to a lesser degree, disparities in health in hopes of resolving our paradoxical crisis of health care and health. Donald Berwick, Thomas Nolan, and John Whittington (2008) have articulated "the triple aim" for improving the health care system: (1) "improving the experience of care," (2) "improving the health of populations," and (3) "reducing per capita costs (i.e., expenditures) of health care." However, their ideas for policy change, including greater linkages to social services, are largely oriented toward health policy of the type embodied in the Affordable Care Act (and discussed in chapter 2). Their ideas cannot be extended to the broad range of nonhealth aspects of social policy emphasized in part II of this book. Elizabeth Bradley and her colleagues (2011) and Elizabeth Bradley and Lauren Taylor (2013) use the term "American Health Care Paradox" for what I term our "paradoxical crisis of health care and health." They also identify a U.S. deficiency in social expenditures as playing some role in it (as discussed further in chapter 9). But again, they propose resolving the paradox largely through the health care system and linking it better to social services; Bradley and Taylor (2013, 174) explicitly eschew as politically and economically

unfeasible "the expansion of social services" or a "transfer [of] funding from health care to social service provisions." Finally, the Robert Wood Johnson Foundation has been moving toward a policy of promoting a "culture of health," as yet only vaguely defined, and has used the title "Beyond the Affordable Care Act: Achieving Real Improvements in Americans' Health" (Williams, McClellan, and Rivlin 2010). Though these researchers recognize large social disparities in health and their roots in a broad range of social determinants, like Bradley and Taylor, they also largely advocate for solutions based in a combination of health and social services, eschewing a focus on disparities or on the key social policies (for example, education, income, civil rights, macroeconomics) that drive population health and its disparities, and hence any demand-side policy. This book argues that we must look to exactly these policy areas for an effective demand-side policy that can significantly improve population health and reduce health care expenditures.

Chapter 2

1. Jonathan Oberlander (2011) provides a nice historical overview of the legislative path to the ACA and explains how and why it compromised the act's potency. The Supreme Court decision upholding the ACA further weakened the impact of its proposed expansion of Medicaid, as has the failure of many states to enact the Medicaid expansion and/or insurance exchanges. And the degree to which the uninsured will opt to buy the insurance available to them remains an open question, though initial results are positive, especially in states that have entered vigorously into both Medicaid expansion and state-run insurance exchanges. The achievement of other less central elements of the ACA is similarly uncertain. See also Kingdon (1984/2011).
2. Much of this section derives heavily from the work of Jacob Hacker (2002), who is in turn indebted to Gøsta Esping-Andersen (1990) and Richard Titmuss (1958).
3. See Quadagno (2006) for an excellent sociological history of opposition to health care and insurance reform in America in the twentieth century; for a discussion of current obstacles to reform, see Fuchs and Milstein (2011).
4. For example, a reasonably representative longitudinal study by Catherine Ross and John Mirowsky (2000, abstract, 151–52) found "that persons with private insurance do not differ significantly from the uninsured in their self-reported health, physical functioning, or number of chronic conditions, whereas persons with public insurance report significantly worse health . . . insurance does not mediate any associations between SES and health . . . but does reduce difficulties in paying medical bills, and Medicaid is associated with more doctor visits and prescription drugs." This is generally consistent with the conclusion of thorough reviews by Helen Levy and David Meltzer (2001, 2008): "Many of the studies claiming to show a causal effect of health insurance on health do not do so convincingly." However, they appropriately also conclude that some studies provide "convincing evidence . . . that health insurance can improve the health measure of some population subgroups" (Levy and Meltzer 2008, 399), perhaps most notably studies showing that early expansions of Medicaid improved women's and children's

health (Currie and Gruber 1996a, 1996b). These studies also note that such expenditures (an estimated $840,000 per infant life saved) might not be cost-effective, an issue also raised by Levy and Meltzer.

5. Brook et al. (2006), 3.
6. Michalopoulos et al. (2012), 764.
7. Baicker et al. (2013), 1713.
8. Courtmanche and Zapata (2014); Sommers, Long, and Baicker (2014); Van der Wees, Zaslavsky, and Ayanian (2013).
9. Sommers, Long, and Baiker (2014), 589–92.
10. This statement reflects: (1) the estimates of a range of economists prior to the passage of ACA (*The Economists' Voice* 2010); (2) the estimates of the Office of the Actuary of the Centers for Medicare and Medicaid Services (CMS) just after the passage of ACA (Sisko et al. 2010; for the most recent estimates, see Hartman et al. 2013), which project a modest increase in spending due to ACA; and (3) estimates of the Congressional Budget Office (CBO) and the Joint Committee on Taxation (JCT) that are similar to the CMS estimates (Banthin and Masi 2013). Proponents of reform tend to predict reductions in spending due to ACA, while opponents predict increases. Very recently, some have suggested that decreases in the rate of increased health care spending from 2009 to 2011 (visible in figure 1.1) may reflect structural changes in the health care and insurance system attributable to ACA and other forces rather than merely the effects of the Great Recession (Cutler and Sahni 2013; Ryu et al. 2013). However, neither CMS nor CBO/JCT has substantially reduced long-term estimates of growth to reflect this possibility, and others attribute at least 70 percent of the recent slowdown in health spending growth to the Great Recession (Dranove, Garthwaite, and Ody 2014). It is notable in figure 1.1 that other nations show very similar leveling-off increases in health expenditures as a percentage of GDP, despite having varying systems of health insurance and care and despite not having implemented major health care reform. Forthcoming data for 2012 and beyond will be necessary to have increased confidence that ACA will significantly reduce health spending, as much as I and many others hope that it may.
11. The problems and uncertainties regarding the impact of EHRs on quality of care, health, and health spending and costs have been discussed in both the popular press (for example, see Milt Freudenheim, "Digitizing Health Records, Before It Was Cool," *New York Times*, January 15, 2012) and scientific publications (Black et al. 2011; Chaudhry et al. 2006; Kellermann and Jones 2013), prompting even the strongest HER proponents to urge care, caution, and patience in our expectations for and implementation of EHRs (Blumenthal 2013; Kellermann and Jones 2013). In any event, large impacts of EHRs on quality of care, health, and cost reduction appear, at best, some years away.
12. The ACA also includes provisions (such as accountable care organizations that try to improve population health by means other than medical care and in cooperation with private and public organizations other than health care providers. This idea also has promise, but operates at the level of the catchment area of health care systems. Thus, it will be difficult for such provisions to affect broader state and national policies of the type that are

most consequential for health and which are discussed in part II, especially chapter 7.

13. David Cutler (2014), a leading health economist and adviser to the Obama administration on the Affordable Care Act, has recently published an optimistic assessment of ACA's potential to use quality improvement to reduce or even halt the increase in health costs and expenditures while also improving population health. The key levers that he examines are: (1) increasing the use of information technology and EHRs; (2) moving away from fee-for-service payment to prospective or bundled payments; and (3) making substantial organizational change in the "internal structures [of health organizations and the larger system] to deliver higher quality, lower cost care" (Cutler 2014, 135). Cutler provides a nuanced discussion of how all this could unfold over the next couple of decades, but also of the many potential problems and pitfalls along the way. Thus, again, we can all hope for the best, but our expectations regarding ACA's impact on the quality and cost-effectiveness of care, expenditures for health care and insurance, and population health must be more modest and realistic.

Chapter 3

1. This book, like most health policy and health care reforms, focuses on physical health but also includes mental health. Although most of the arguments and evidence discussed apply to mental as well as physical health, I recognize that there are special issues in the etiology, course, and treatment of any given mental disease or mental health problem.
2. See Cutler (2004), Cutler, Rosen, and Vijan (2006), and Murphy and Topel (2006) for influential analyses of the health and economic value of health care.
3. For the decades of the 1960s through the 1990s, David Cutler and his colleagues (2006) estimate the average per person cost, in constant 2002 dollars, of a one-year increase in life expectancy at birth and at ages fifteen, forty-five, and sixty-five. They show that the per person cost per year increases with both age and every decade since the 1970s. Gains in life expectancy are now more likely to be made at old age, but the cost of each year of increased life at age sixty-five more than tripled from the 1970s, when it was $46,800, to the 1990s, when it was $145,000. Cutler and his colleagues conclude that "the former amount certainly reflects a good value, but the latter fails to meet many cost-benefit criteria" (924). These estimates assume that 50 percent of improvements in life expectancy are due to health care. As we will see, that is arguably an upper-bound estimate, and the declining cost-effectiveness of health care would worsen as the proportion of gains in life expectancy attributable to medical care declined below 50 percent.
4. This is one form of what Amos Tversky and Daniel Kahneman (1974) refer to as the *availability* heuristic or bias, one of several broad heuristics or biases used by people in their everyday decisions or causal inferences. This leads to outcomes that are not rational, logical, or empirically valid. Much research by Kahneman and Tversky and others indicates that because dramatic or prominent events or persons are more easily thought of or available when

we try to pull together information in our mind, we are likely to overweight them relative to less dramatic or prominent events when we make decisions or draw inferences. See also Kahneman (2011) for a recent and accessible discussion of availability and other biases in thinking and decision-making.

5. We may also tend to embellish our memories of dramatic events over time. A physician reading a draft of this book felt that the speed of response of my blood pressure to medication that I remember is probably not possible. So our attributions errors and biases may grow with time.
6. Much of the remainder of this chapter is covered in greater detail and with many more references in House (2002).
7. For an account that is both scholarly and readable, see Paul Starr's (1982) book on the development of the medical profession and the medical-biotechnology complex over the course of American history, especially from 1850 to 1980. George Rosen (1958) provides the fullest coverage of the development of public health, with the period since the mid-twentieth century covered in an excellent introductory essay by Elizabeth Fee (1993) that is included in a later (1993) edition of Rosen's volume.
8. Quoted in Rosen (1979).
9. Quoted in Bloom (1990), 1–2. See Bloom (2002) for a fuller history of social medicine and medical sociology.
10. Flexner (1910).
11. As discussed at greater length in chapter 6, behavioral science was added to some medical school curricula in the 1960s and 1970s, and very recently the Medical College Admission Test (MCAT) has decided to include questions on social and behavioral science in response to recommendations for broadening premedical and medical education. Such efforts as yet do not even approximate what Virchow had in mind in 1848.
12. The concept and theory of the epidemiologic transition was developed by Abdel Omran (1971).
13. Robert Aronowitz (1998) provides a good discussion of the concept of risk factors and its development. It should be noted that the causation of infectious disease is often complex and multifactorial, as in our discussion of the decline of tuberculosis and other infectious diseases later in this chapter, and that some infections, such as AIDS, Lyme disease if not treated properly, and hepatitis C, become chronic diseases.
14. See Dawber (1980) for an overview and appreciation of the first several decades of the Framingham Study, which continues to this day.
15. See Surgeon General's Advisory Committee on Smoking and Health (1964) and later editions and updates of the Surgeon General's Report (Center for Public Program Evaluation 2011).
16. For an overview of these studies at of the beginning of the twentieth century, see House (2002) and Berkman and Kawachi (2000).
17. The development of this evidence is elaborated somewhat in House (2002) and in greater detail in Taylor, Repetti, and Seeman (1997).
18. This general idea was first noted by Thomas McKeown and Reginald Record (1962) but developed more fully in McKeown (1976), the original source for figure 3.3. In later works, McKeown (1979, 1988) increasingly, and appropriately, emphasized that medical care does more to alleviate the pain and suf-

fering associated with morbidity and mortality than to prevent or cure morbidity or reduce mortality. So analyses of mortality probably provide a lower-bound estimate of the impact of medical care on health more broadly.

19. McKinlay and McKinlay (1977).
20. Simon Szreter (2002) argues for attributing a greater role in the decline of tuberculosis to public health measures. James Colgrove (2002) and Tommy Bengtsson (2001) provide measured overviews of the disputes and draw conclusions similar to those expressed here.
21. Bunker, Frazier, and Mosteller (1994).
22. Michael McGinnis, Pamela Williams-Russo, and James Knickman (2002) suggest that the figure should be as low as 10 percent for medical care, but up to 30 percent for genetic factors. The proportional effects assigned to medical care versus other factors are also hard to estimate with great precision because the line between medical care and other factors is often blurred. For example, when physicians individually or as professional societies recommend the use of seatbelts or other means of reducing accidental injury and death, is this medical care or just part of a broader societal effort to reduce accidental injury and death? The point here is not to determine the exact percentage of the variance in morbidity and mortality attributable to medical care, but rather to show that, while the estimates range from 10 percent to perhaps as high as 50 percent, most put it at 10 to 30 percent (that is, with a mode of 20 percent plus or minus 10 percent), which is far below the assumption that health care is the main or sole determinant of health underlying both our conventional wisdom and public policy regarding health.
23. This argument was perhaps first made by Robert Evans and Greg Stoddart (1994) in the context of a broader argument for giving social determinants of health a more central place in health science and policy.
24. Medical care practitioners and systems do play a role in preventing as well as treating disease. Their inoculation (that is, vaccination or immunization) of their patients against disease is one form of primary prevention (see figures 3.6 and 3.7), and they can also discuss with their patients ways to promote healthful conditions of life and work. Screening and early detection of disease is another major activity of the medical care system. Although screening is often termed "secondary prevention," it is really just earlier detection of disease rather than prevention of its onset. Moreover, the costs and benefits of screening are highly variable and often controversial, as seen in ongoing discussions and changing recommendations. For example, measuring blood pressure and analyzing blood samples for lipids and sugar are medical procedures that are clearly and almost universally desirable and useful; mammography is desirable and useful only for many people, but not all; and screening for prostate cancer via physical examination or PSA (prostate specific antigen) tests is increasingly seen as neither desirable nor useful.

Chapter 4

1. Note that (maximum) life *span* for a population refers here and generally to the (maximum) number of years any member of that population can live. Life *expectancy* refers to the number of years that a median person—or 50

percent of a population—is expected to live from a given age (birth, age twenty-five, age sixty-five, or some other age *x*). Life expectancy reflects the application of age-specific mortality rates—either those currently observed or those projected for the future—to each year of life after the given age. Thus, although the human life span may have changed little, if at all, over the past 250 years, human life expectancy has increased dramatically. Some argue that life span may increase, especially as a population grows older, though the evidence for this is usually based on research in nonhuman populations (mainly fruit flies and rodents) or on extrapolation from the fact that there is as yet no clear limit on human life *expectancy*. No one contests, however, that no human has been authenticated to have lived more than 122.5 years, a record attained almost two decades ago. And the apparent leveling, or even reduction, of mortality rates in very old humans (centenarians) compared with mortality rates for those who are just old (noncentenarians) most likely reflects the unusual robustness or lack of frailty in those who make it to 100, what social scientists refer to as a "selection bias" or "selection problem." Wikipedia provides balanced and scholarly discussions of both life expectancy and life span, and Jonathan Silvertown (2013) engagingly discusses these issues across species, historical times, and ages of the life course. James Vaupel (2010) represents probably the strongest and most credible proponent of the view that there may be no clear limit on human life span. Recent trends suggest that the growth of life expectancy in some of the longest-lived human populations (for example, Japanese and Swiss women) may be slowing (see figures 1.2 to 1.6), as would be expected as these populations begin to approach the biological limits on the human life span.

2. This and the next two paragraphs draw heavily on Coale (1974), which remains a scholarly yet readable account of the growth of human population up to the early part of the second half of the twentieth century.
3. Again, as discussed in chapter 3, note 22, the specific percentage attributable to "medical care" varies depending on what is included under that rubric. The 20 percent plus or minus 10 percent estimate derives largely from considering therapeutic medical care, though it probably does not include the efforts of doctors or physician groups to increase vaccinations and persuade people to drive safely, use seat belts, stop smoking, and lose weight. With the exception of vaccinations, such efforts are generally not very effective anyway. Widespread vaccinations remain challenging, even in the United States.
4. Figures 4.1 and 4.2 are stylized constructions by the author, though they approximate actual data. The concept of rectangularization of the mortality or survival curve of a population was developed by biologists (see, for example, Comfort 1956, 1964) and extended to human populations by a number of demographers, especially in France (for example, Levy 1996; Martel and Bourbeau 2003) and the United States (Cheung et al. 2005; Manton and Tolley 1991; Wilmoth and Horiuchi 1999). The idea of the compression of morbidity (and functional limitations) is largely attributable to James Fries (1980, 2000) and his colleagues (Fries and Crapo 1981). These ideas have provoked extensive debate over how fixed and finite the human life span is: Do improvements in life expectancy (and the incidence and prevalence of disease and functional limitations) involve rectangularization and compression rela-

tive to a finite limit? Or can improvements continue indefinitely? Since Fries introduced his ideas, there has been considerable debate as to whether compression of morbidity and functional limitations has occurred or been observed. If the answer is yes, then it is possible to add not only "years to life" but also "life to years" (Hauser 1953). That is, the number of healthy and active years can increase as life expectancy increases, rather than just the number of years spent with worsening illness and disability, as others have argued (Schneider and Brody 1983; Verbrugge 1984). The empirical answer discussed in this chapter is maybe yes, and maybe no.

5. A similar argument was made by David Kindig and John Mullahy (2010).
6. Samuel Preston and Michael Haines (1991) make an argument of this type with respect to individual income and occupation in relation to child mortality in the United States in the late nineteenth and very early twentieth centuries. However, they also note that race and other socioeconomic factors were quite important—such as being unemployed, renting versus owning, being a laborer, and being illiterate or not speaking English—as was the average income of the state of residence. Many of these factors are consequential in developing countries today, especially maternal education and literacy. Preston and Haines also show that occupations became more consequential in urban areas, and that occupation was much more clearly consequential at the beginning of the twentieth century in England and Wales, which were much more industrialized and urbanized. Others have argued that socioeconomic differences were smaller in pre-twentieth-century England (Razzell and Spence 2006). Analyses in Sweden find that socioeconomic differentials are largely a post–World War II phenomenon (Bengtsson and Dribe 2011), while in the Netherlands a socioeconomic gradient was evident before the twentieth century (van Poppel, Jennissen, and Mandemakers 2009). It appears that socioeconomic disparities are variable across time and place but have been evident in many places and times, with factors like occupation and income generally becoming more important as populations have become more urban and industrial rather than rural and agricultural. For present purposes, it is clear that socioeconomic differences in health were sizable and pervasive within and across major industrialized and urbanized nations by the middle of the twentieth century, yet not widely recognized or attended to.
7. Freeman, Levine, and Reeder (1972), 501–2. This view was part of a failure in some quarters to see poverty and inequality in American society. That failure had been breached on a broader front by the publication of Michael Harrington's (1962) *The Other America,* which many observers credited with stimulating President Lyndon Johnson's War on Poverty and related Great Society programs, including Medicare and Medicaid.
8. Douglas Black et al. (1982), 39.
9. Ibid., 11. The Reagan administration similarly buried the 1985 "Report of the Secretary's [of Health and Human Services] Task Force on Black and Minority Health," which did not receive the kind of nongovernmental resurrection that the Black Report did.
10. Pappas et al. (1993).
11. Wilkins, Adams, and Brancker (1989).

12. Keynes (1923), ch. 3.
13. For more detail on all of these ACL data and replication of our findings in the National Health Interview Survey, see House et al. (1990), House et al. (1994), and House, Lantz, and Herd (2005); also see our website at: http://www.isr.umich.edu/acl/. See Zimmer and House (2003) and Herd, Goesling, and House (2007) for the differential effects of education and income. A large body of work overviewed by Robert Hummer and Elaine Hernandez (2013) shows large and growing educational differences in levels of mortality and life expectancy. For example, at age twenty-five, female college graduates in the United States can expect to live a dozen years longer than women who did not graduate from high school, with a similar difference of thirteen to sixteen years among men (Rostron, Boies, and Arias 2010). Dustin Brown and his colleagues (2012) show that the more-educated manifest not only longer life on average but greater rectangularization and compression of mortality.
14. See Newman (2003).
15. Although people's level of education is a function of their parents' socioeconomic position, their childhood health problems, the personal and social contexts in which they grew up, and their genes and unborn capabilities, Hummer and Hernandez (2013) show that such factors explain relatively little of the educational disparities in health over the life course.
16. Drawing on threads from earlier work, Bruce Link and Jo Phelan have developed the theory and evidence for "fundamental cause" theory, including the ideas and evidence in this and the prior paragraph (Link and Phelan 1995, 2000; Phelan et al. 2004; Phelan, Link, and Tehranifar 2010).
17. See Lantz et al. (1998) for our ACL data and references noted in previous and succeeding notes for other data. Note that health is promoted by moderate levels of drinking alcohol and eating and by maintaining a moderate weight, whereas both low and high levels of drinking and eating and both high and low weight constitute risk factors for health.
18. Studies before and after our ACL study show similar socioeconomic disparities in levels of biomedical as well as behavioral and psychosocial risk factors, as well as similar explanatory power (Lynch et al. 1996; Marmot, Kogevinas, and Elston 1987). Hummer and Hernandez (2013) review a half-dozen more recent studies that show a similar patterning and impact of this wide range of explanatory risk factors. In another recent review, Karen Matthews, Linda Gallo, and Shelley Taylor (2010) draw a more guarded conclusion, but my reading suggests that the studies they review that include larger population-based samples, major health outcomes such as mortality, and a range of psychosocial risk factors are consistent with what is argued here.
19. See Lantz et al. (1998, 2005, 2010) for the supporting ACL data. Note 17 and chapter 3 provide corroborating evidence from other studies. Some recent studies have suggested an explanatory power for health behaviors in relation to mortality that is more in the range of 50 percent in some populations. Our own further analyses (Mehta, House, and Elliott, forthcoming) suggest that the degree to which risky health behaviors explain disparities by both education and income varies for education versus income and over time,

place, and population under study (such as younger working people versus older retired people). The basic point remains that health behaviors alone can only *begin* to explain why we have such large socioeconomic disparities in health.

20. See note 13.
21. See note 4.
22. The definitive evidence of this came from review and analyses of multiple data sets by Vicki Freedman and her colleagues (2004).
23. Comparative evidence indicates that the pervasive mortality and life expectancy disadvantage of the U.S. population relative to other comparably developed nations diminishes slightly with increasing age, and much more dramatically after age seventy-five, with the United States among the nations with the best life expectancy after age eighty-five (Ho and Preston 2010).
24. See also Schoeni et al. (2005).
25. See House et al. (2005) for a fuller discussion of these data and the larger ACL study. The same researchers who identified declines in old-age disability over the same period, from the mid-1980s to the beginning of the twenty-first century, also found that such declines were much greater at higher socioeconomic levels (Schoeni et al. 2005).
26. See Martin and Schoeni (2014) for similar findings from repeated cross-sectional studies. It is too early to know definitively why this is the case. There are both differences between individuals in these two age cohorts (fifty-five to sixty-nine in 1986 versus fifty-five to sixty-nine in 2001–2002) and differences in the societal environments in which they transitioned from late middle age (fifty-five to sixty-nine) to early and middle old age (seventy to eighty-four), the prosperous and relatively peaceful era of 1986–2001 versus the economically and internationally troubled past decade. Initial analyses of our ACL data suggest several ways in which those age fifty-five to sixty-nine in 2001–2002 manifested greater levels of psychosocial risk factors for health than those of the same age in 1986: they were heavier and more likely to be obese, they were more likely to have experienced negative life events (especially separation and divorce), and they were less likely to be moderate drinkers. But as they transitioned to early and middle old age (seventy to eighty-four), they also clearly lived in times that were more difficult at all socioeconomic levels.
27. See Dow and Rehkopf (2010).

Chapter 5

1. Robert Hummer and his colleagues (2013) provide an overview of national statistics on the racial-ethnic and gender disparities in mortality and life expectancy, especially in their table 9.3. Although women live longer than men and have had lower rates of most life-threatening disorders, they have higher rates of acute conditions and many debilitating but not life-threatening diseases, such as arthritis and osteoporosis (Rieker and Bird 2000; Verbrugge and Wingard 1987). As discussed in chapter 1 and further in this chapter, the

female advantage in life expectancy in the United States has been eroding over the past three decades (see also Rieker, Bird, and Lang 2010).

2. There are vast literatures on the social construction of race, and also on the relations between race and genetics. David Williams (1994) and Thomas LaVeist (2005) provide an entrée into the "social constructionist" perspective. Francis Collins (2004), Michael Fine, Said Ibrahim, and Stephen Thomas (2005), Neil Pearce and his colleagues (2004), and Pamela Sankar and her colleagues (2004) all recognize some genetic differences between races, but tend to concur that there is little current evidence for a significant role of genetics in explaining broad racial disparities in health.
3. Robert Hummer and Juanita Chinn (2011) estimate that "even weakly measured" socioeconomic factors account for the "majority" (close to 70 percent) of the racial differences in mortality and life expectancy in the United States.
4. Smedley, Stith, and Nelson (2003).
5. See Pascoe and Smart Richman (2009) for a thorough review of 134 studies linking perceived discrimination to mental and physical health and extensive analyses and discussion of causality, the pathways for such effects, and possible moderating factors. See also Williams and Mohammed (2009), Williams, Neighbors, and Jackson (2003), and Clark et al. (1999).
6. Williams and Chiquita Collins (2013) and Delores Acevedo-Garcia and colleagues (2003) conceptualize and empirically review the adverse impacts of residential segregation on health. See also Kawachi and Berkman (2003) for more general discussion of how neighborhoods affect health.
7. For evidence that racial segregation and associated neighborhood factors may explain why African Americans continue to have a higher prevalence of hypertension than whites (even when in treatment) despite the elimination of racial disparities in the awareness of and treatment for hypertension, see Morenoff et al. (2007).
8. Strawbridge et al. (1997); Hummer et al. (1999a); Musick, House, and Williams (2004).
9. See McGuire and Miranda (2008) on racial-ethnic differences in depression and Hummer et al. (1999b) and Cho et al. (2004) on the Latino "paradox." The nature and degree of such differences often vary across health measures and populations studied, and the reasons for these differences are complex. The point here is simply that race-ethnicity may not generally predict health as strongly and consistently as socioeconomic position does, but it still constitutes an additional dimension of social disparities in health.
10. World Health Organization (2013).
11. See recent reports from the National Research Council (2011a, 2011c) and the National Research Council and Institute of Medicine (2013) for the best and fullest analyses and discussions to date of the possible reasons for the worsening mortality and life expectancy of American women.
12. David Kindig and Erika Cheng (2013) find absolutely declining female life expectancy in more than 40 percent of U.S. counties, and those counties are concentrated in geographical areas with generally lower socioeconomic levels. Jennifer Montez and her colleagues (2011), Jay Olshansky and his colleagues (2012), and Jennifer Montez and Anna Zajacova (2013b) show that

white women with less than a high school education have manifested decreasing life expectancy; Montez and Zajacova (2013a) attribute this decline about equally to smoking (and other health behaviors) and women's employment, which is to say, their lack thereof and the associated socioeconomic disadvantages.

13. These effects have been conceptualized, empirically documented, and referred to as "weathering" by Arline Geronimus (1991, 2001; Geronimus, Bound et al. 2001; Geronimus, Hicken et al. 2006; Geronimus, Hicken, Keene et al. 2010).
14. See Ailshire and House (2011) for a fuller exposition and analysis of the trends discussed here and shown in figure 5.3.
15. I know of no precise estimates of the degree to which gains in life expectancy over the past couple of centuries have come primarily for those disadvantaged in terms of socioeconomic position, race-ethnicity, and gender. However, we do know that for women the life expectancy of the longest-lived 20 percent of the American population changed only slightly over the twentieth century, while that of the shortest-lived 20 percent grew from less than twenty years to almost seventy-five (Fischer and Hout 2006, figure 4.2) . This increase in life expectancy reflected massive declines in infant and child mortality from infectious disease and in childbirth-associated mortality in women. But it undoubtedly reflected the closing of socioeconomic and racial-ethnic disparities as well.

Chapter 6

1. The exact role of fluoride and the importance of different sources of fluoride cannot be precisely estimated. The importance of fluoride toothpaste is suggested by the widespread nature of the decline: dental health has improved in areas both with and without fluoridated water or salt (Brown, Wall, and Lazar 2000).
2. Richard W. Valachovic, Executive Director of the American Dental Education Association, "Current Demographics and Future Trends of the Dentist Workforce," presentation to the "U.S. Oral Health Workforce in the Coming Decade" workshop, Institute of Medicine, February 9, 2009, available at: http://www.iom.edu/~/media/Files/Activity%20Files/Workforce/oralhealthworkforce/2009-Feb-09/1%20-%20Valachovic.ashx. It should be noted that the number of dentists has declined despite substantial efforts to promote discretionary cosmetic forms of dental care.
3. For example, a meta-analysis by Lee Goldman and Francis Cook (1984) attributes 54 percent of the decline in cardiovascular disease to changes in lifestyle and 40 percent to medical intervention. Pamela Sytkowski, William Kannel, and Ralph D'Agostino (1990, 1638) conclude that, "although improved treatment methods and better prevention may have contributed to the decline in [cardiovascular] mortality, our study and others suggest that risk factor modification has played an important part." Using a quantitative model, Maria Hunink and her colleagues (1997) attribute a greater influence to treatment in their suggestion that the impact of reduced risk factors operates equally to prevent disease incidence and prevent progression to fatality

among those with disease. However, using a similar model in England and Wales, Belgin Unal, Julia Alison Critchley, and Simon Capewell (2004) attribute 60 percent of reduced incidence of CVD to risk factor change, especially smoking, and 40 percent to medical treatment. A recent careful and comprehensive review over time and nations concludes: "Changes in risk factors may explain from 44 percent to 76 percent of declining CHD (coronary heart disease) mortality and treatments may explain approximately 23 percent to 47 percent. . . . Economic analyses suggest that primary prevention [prior to medical treatment] in individuals is cost-effective, and in whole populations, it may be cost-saving" (Ford and Capewell 2011, 12, 16).

4. Data from Wikipedia, which draws from data of the National Highway Traffic Safety Administration. There has been less analysis than one might expect of the causes of declines in highway accident deaths, but what analysis there is largely confirms the importance of road and vehicle design factors, restrictions on young drivers, and attempts to reduce drunk driving and improve driver training (Robertson 1996, 2006).
5. This information derives from NIH, Office of Budget (various years).
6. See National Research Council and Institute of Medicine (2013, 8, 286–89) for this recommendation to NIH "or another appropriate entity."
7. Gillum et al. (2011).
8. See Boardman, Daw, and Freese (2013) for an excellent discussion of the ways in which the social environment shapes the expression and effects of genes on health, and vice versa.
9. My characterization of modern medical education derives from a review of web postings on the general state of medical education as well as of the admission requirements and curricula of specific medical schools. It should be noted that the Association of American Medical Colleges (AAMC) is making a substantial revision in the Medical College Admission Test that will go into effect in 2015 (AAMC 2012). The MCAT, which essentially eliminated content outside of biological, physical, chemical, and mathematical science in 1977, is introducing sections on the psychological, social, and biological foundations of behavior and on critical analysis and reasoning, each of which will constitute almost 25 percent of the test; the remaining half will be devoted in equal portions to the biological and biochemical foundations of living systems and to the chemical and physical foundations of biological systems. The social science quarter of the test is heavily weighted, however, toward psychology (60 percent) and biology (10 percent); the rest (30 percent) is focused on sociology. One undergraduate course in psychology and one in sociology are recommended, though not required, as preparation, compared with a suggestion to take two sequential courses in each of biology, chemistry, organic chemistry, and physics, plus one course in biochemistry. The major aim of the social and psychological sciences is making physicians better clinicians. About half of all premedical students (both applicants and accepted students) still major in biological sciences, and only one-sixth major in the social sciences or humanities; another one-sixth major in other natural or health sciences, and one-sixth in all other areas.
10. See National Research Council (2011b) for an overview of the current nature and penetration of HIAs in the United States and recommendations for stan-

dardizing HIA practice and using it more widely. Expanding the consideration of health in EIAs is one recommendation. The Robert Wood Johnson Foundation and the PEW Charitable Trusts have jointly sponsored an ongoing effort to promote and fund HIAs, mostly at the local level but also regarding aspects of major national policies such as the farm bill.

11. Cited by Pekka Puska and Timo Ståhl (2010, 320), who overview the Finnish and EU experience with HiAP.
12. See Ståhl et al. (2006) on the Finnish and European experience; for the ongoing California efforts, see the Health in All Policies Task Force website at: http://www.sgc.ca.gov/s_hiap.php.
13. See Robert Wood Johnson Foundation Commission to Build a Healthier America (2009). At the national level, elements of HiAP are incorporated into the Partnership for Sustainable Communities Program of the Environmental Protection Agency and the Departments of Transportation and Housing and Urban Development, and in the National Prevention Council mandated in the Affordable Care Act of 2010.
14. Acheson et al. (1998).
15. Mackenbach (2011).

Chapter 7

1. Allan Brandt (2007) and Richard Kluger (1997) provide major histories of the rise and fall of cigarette smoking that focus on the great lengths (ultimately largely unsuccessful) to which tobacco companies went to deter effective regulation of tobacco in the last half of the twentieth century.
2. For example, medical and public health scientists tend to attribute the problem to broader agricultural production policies (see, for example, Franck, Grandi, and Eisenberg [2013] and the popular writer Michael Pollan [2006]), while economists favor explanations related to the intermediate processing and sales of food and to consumer choices, such as eating out more, perhaps especially at fast-food outlets (Alston, Okrent, and Parks 2012; Alston, Sumner, and Vosti 2008; Cutler, Glaeser, and Shapiro 2003; Okrent and Alston 2012). All would agree that changes in subsidies and taxes on different kinds of food production, processing, marketing, and consumption could measurably affect the amount and type of food consumed, and hence both obesity and health more generally. Such policy changes are likely to be even harder to achieve, however, than the regulation of tobacco; witness the implosion of Mayor Michael Bloomberg's effort to limit the size of higher-calorie sodas sold in New York City convenience stores.
3. See, for example, American Public Health Association (2007) and Raynault and Christopher (2013) on the negative health impacts of transportation policies beyond reductions in physical activity, such as motor vehicle accidents and environmental pollution. At this point, however, our understanding of the health impact of particular transportation policies and practices is more intuitive than grounded in research, though the body of such research is growing.
4. Supplemented by more recent basic research and policy evaluation, much of what follows draws heavily on Robert Schoeni and colleagues (2008), who

extensively consider the health impacts of these policies (along with a more specific policy, the welfare reform of the late 1990s, that cuts across all of these areas and others).

5. This influential formulation was developed by the political scientist John Kingdon (1984/2011).
6. This discussion draws heavily on the work of Jonathan Oberlander (2011, 2012a, 2012b). Simon Haeder (2012) provides a good overview of the recent literature on how and why the ACA came to pass in the form that it did and future prospects for its implementation. It should be noted that after the failure of comprehensive health care reform in the first term of the Clinton administration, Senator Edward Kennedy of Massachusetts, with considerable support from Hillary Rodham Clinton, worked with Republican Senator Orrin Hatch of Utah in Bill Clinton's second term to pass, in 1997, the state-based Children's Health Insurance Program (CHIP, previously known as SCHIP). The CHIP program was expanded to ultimately cover about 8 million lower-income children. As in the 1960s, this program dealt with one impoverished portion of the population, leaving the situation of the non-poor, non-elderly, and many poor adults to be addressed in the 2010 ACA. (For a reasonable overview of CHIP's history, see "State Children's Health Insurance Program," Wikipedia, http://en.wikipedia.org/wiki/State_Children%27s_Health_Insurance_Program.)
7. Austin Bradford Hill (1965), one of the pioneering epidemiologists in identifying the health hazards of cigarette smoking, provided a very good statement of how a broad range of evidence can accumulate, even in the absence of experimental studies on humans, to provide a strong basis for causal inference. R. A. Fisher, a population geneticist and the father of modern experimental design and statistical analysis of experimental data, and a cigarette smoker, went to his grave at age seventy-two arguing, with support from tobacco companies, that the lack of experimental evidence made it impossible to conclude that cigarette smoking caused lung cancer and other fatal diseases; see "Ronald Fisher," Wikipedia, http://en.wikipedia.org/wiki/Ronald_Fisher. Hill, who had tuberculosis during World War I military service, was initially a smoker but gave it up as a result of his research; he died in 1991 at age ninety-five. His collaborator, Richard Doll, similarly quit smoking, then lived to ninety-three. See "Sir Austin Bradford Hill," Science Museum History of Medicine, http://www.sciencemuseum.org.uk/broughttolife/people/austinhill.aspx.
8. International comparative data on spending and education skills drawn from OECD (2013a). For data on government spending on education and other sectors in the United States, see "Government Spending in the U.S.," available at: www.usgovernmentspending.com.
9. For reviews of the findings on education discussed in this section, see Cutler and Lleras-Muney (2008) and Hummer and Hernandez (2013). For a similar review of early childhood education's effects on health and other indicators of human development, see Keating and Simonton (2008). Pamela Herd and her colleagues (2007) show that education plays a primary role in preventing the onset of health problems, while income plays a primary role in slowing the progression of health problems up to and including death. James Riley

(2001) provides an overview of the effects of education within and across the nations of the world.

10. The estimates of the economic costs and value of increases in life expectancy due to postsecondary student financial aid derive from Cutler and Adriana Lleras-Muney (2008), extrapolating from the work of Susan Dynarski (2003). Ezra Golberstein, Richard Hirth, and Paula Lantz (2012) provide a congruent estimate of 0.2 to 0.4 quality-adjusted years of life (valued at $26,000 to $49,000) from an additional year of education. The estimates of the costs in terms of lifetime medical spending for an additional year of life expectancy are from Cutler, Rosen, and Vijan (2006).
11. This estimate is also from Cutler and Lleras-Muney (2008).
12. See OECD (2013b).
13. See Herd, Goesling, and House (2007), Herd, House, and Schoeni (2008), and Herd, Schoeni, and House (2008).
14. For literature reviews and new empirical evidence regarding SSI and EITC, see Herd, House, and Schoeni (2008), Herd, Schoeni, and House (2008b), Hoynes, Miller, and Simon (2012), and Evans and Garthwaite (2014). Positive health effects have also been shown for the introduction and increase of food stamps through the Supplemental Nutrition Assistance Program, which is partially a targeted nutrition assistance program and partially a general income support program, as it frees up the other income of poor people for other uses that may be beneficial to health (Almond, Hoynes, and Schanzenbach 2011).
15. See Arno et al. (2011).
16. The initial study was conducted by Paul Taubman and Robin Sickles (1983) and the later one by Herd, House, and Schoeni (2008) and Herd, Schoeni, and House (2008b).
17. On the Mexican program, see Fernald, Gertler, and Neufeld (2008); on the Ecuador income support program, see Paxson and Schady (2007); on South African old-age pensions, see Case (2004).
18. See Sullivan and von Wachter (2009a, 2009b) on the effects of job loss on future earnings and life expectancy and the degree to which loss of earnings and income produces or accounts for the health effects of job loss discussed here. See also Kessler, Turner, and House (1988) for analogous evidence regarding mental health and self-rated health.
19. See Tapia Granados and Diez Roux (2009). José Tapia Granados and his colleagues (2014) have recently shown for the United States over the last several decades that individuals suffering unemployment experience major adverse health effects, but that the health of those who do *not* directly experience unemployment improves.
20. Christopher Ruhm (2008) and José Tapia Granados (2005a, 2005b, 2008) provide evidence and explanation for all of this across multiple historical periods and nations.
21. Ruhm (2008).
22. See Almond, Chay, and Greenstone (2006).
23. Most of the rest of this section derives from Kaplan, Ranjit, and Burgard (2008).
24. Case (2004).

25. See Johnson (2011).
26. See Smedley, Stith, and Nelson (2003) for striking evidence in the area of health care.
27. See Massey and Denton (1993) on the general problem of persisting de facto segregation, which has been also still de jure in certain ways.
28. See Morenoff et al. (2007) regarding neighborhoods and blood pressure, and Hicken et al. (2014) regarding the role of vigilance in blood pressure. For reviews of evidence on the health effects of actual, perceived, and anticipated discrimination more generally, see Williams, Neighbors, and Jackson (2003), Williams and Mohammed (2009), and Pascoe and Richman (2009).
29. Morenoff et al. (2008) and Fauth and Brookes-Gunn (2008) provide good overviews of research on the impact of neighborhoods on health.
30. See Ludwig et al. (2011) for a recent overview and key results for MTO; for a review of the experience of the first five years, see Kling, Liebman, and Katz (2007); see also Sanbonmatsu et al. (2011).

Chapter 8

1. Michael Grossman was responsible, in the 1970s, for the seminal consolidation of this idea of human health as a critical human capital element of economic productivity; he also saw health as a consumption as well as an investment good. The idea remains a central foundation of health economics, as can be seen in texts and encyclopedia entries on health economics. For a more recent statement, see Grossman (2000).
2. Nobel Laureate Robert Fogel largely initiated this line of economic thinking, which has been continued by him, his students, and others (see Fogel 2004, 2012; Fogel et al. 2011).
3. For a discussion, see Schoeni et al. (2011, S69), based on the earlier work of Hirth et al. (2000) and Ubel et al. (2003).
4. See Schoeni et al. (2011).
5. Mitra, Findley, and Sambamoorthi (2009).
6. Anderson et al. (2010).
7. Keskimäki, Salinto, and Aro (1995) and Economou, Nikolaou, and Theodossiou (2008).
8. Xu, Nelson, and Berk (2009).
9. Bhattacharya and Sood (2011).
10. This section is based on Michaud et al. (2011).
11. It is difficult to directly compare the research on the impact of health improvements on health care expenditures with discussions and projections of the effects of currently proposed health care and insurance reform on future health care expenditures. The latter are in many ways much more hypothetical than the former, as they rely on projecting at a national level the effects of changes in the health care and insurance system that either have never been tried or have been implemented on only a limited scale. Further, they have not yet been evaluated in full-population projection models of the type used in figures 8.1 to 8.3. As a point of comparison, one of the leading proponents of health care reform (Commonwealth Fund 2013) has very recently projected $2 trillion savings in total national health expenditures over ten years

if a very broad array of health care reforms had all been implemented immediately in 2013—a pretty implausible scenario, both absolutely and relative to the gradual approach that underlies figures 8.2 and 8.3. Even this highly optimistic scenario projects national health expenditures in 2023 of $5.1 trillion, which is $400 billion, or 7 percent, lower than current projections. About half of the total $2 trillion saving over ten years would redound to private employers, households, and state governments, and about half to the federal government. Note that, unlike the numbers in figures 8.1 to 8.3 and the associated text, these numbers are not adjusted for inflation. Overall, the projected savings from improving population health demonstrated in figures 8.1 to 8.3 arguably rival or exceed the savings from the most optimistic scenarios of health care reform in both their magnitude and their likelihood of coming to pass, especially given the inability of previous efforts at health care reform to significantly restrain the growth of health care and insurance spending.

12. Chokshi and Farley (2012).

Chapter 9

1. One may wonder about the role of genetic factors—a major current preoccupation of basic biomedical science—as a determinant of health. For a given individual, and hence in a certain sense for a given population *at a given point in time,* health is clearly influenced by genetic factors, which may account for up to 30 to 40 percent of the variation in the health of individuals over their life courses and in the health of a given population of individuals, again, *at a given point in time.* However, the expression and effects of an organism's genes are heavily influenced by the environment of that organism, and the genetic makeups of individuals and especially populations change very slowly over long periods of time. In contrast, individuals' environments can change quite quickly, either their immediate environment or any new environment to which they move. Therefore, changes in population health over periods of years, decades, or even several centuries are largely a function of changes in environments and their impacts on the development of individuals and populations. McGinnis, Williams-Russo, and Knickman (2002) and Boardman, Daw, and Freese (2013) discuss many of these issues.

   This has certainly been the case for the United States and other developed societies over the past two to three centuries. Modern biomedical science, especially via vaccination and biochemical control of infectious agents such as mosquitoes, played an important role in the initial gains in population health in developing countries in the two to three decades after World War II. But much evidence also suggests a major and probably increasing role for broader patterns of social and economic development in these nations. For a good discussion of changes in the various factors in the improvement of population health over nations and time, see Riley (2001).
2. For data showing generally steady growth in local and state spending from 1900 through about 1970, flat to declining local and state spending thereafter, and not enough new federal spending to offset this decline, see "Government

Spending in the U.S.," available at: http://www.usgovernmentspending.com.

3. The growth of inequality in the United States and much of the world has become an increasing focus of academic and public discourse, with Thomas Piketty's *Capital in the Twenty-First Century* (2014) being the single largest and most important contribution to that discourse to date. In thinking about health, it is not inequality per se that is the crucial issue, but the form that increasing inequality has taken, perhaps especially in the United States: the broad lower half of the socioeconomic distribution is making little progress, or even regressing, in their conditions of life and work and hence in their health. Thus, from one more angle, we see that health policy must become broad social policy, and especially socioeconomic policy. Yet much discussion of inequality fails to consider its connection to health.
4. See Goldin and Katz (2008) and Fischer and Hout (2006) regarding changes in the economy and the growing importance of education. Claude Fischer and Michael Hout also discuss the decline in the minimum wage, which is currently receiving renewed political and policy attention, and the shrinkage of labor unions. For more regarding labor unions, see Rosenfeld (2014). All of these changes contributed to a post-1980 disjunction in the relation between productivity and median earnings or income, which had previously grown together; after 1980, only productivity and the incomes of the higher education and income strata continued to grow, while incomes at or below the median stagnated or even declined in real terms.
5. There is no question that America's mid-twentieth-century epidemic of cigarette smoking has also played a major role in the country's later-twentieth-century population health problems. However, smoking cannot be the whole story and is arguably not even the major part of it. Smoking had its most dramatic impacts on men's health prior to 1980, whereas the period of central concern in this book is the period since 1980. Smoking continues to affect women's health, but again, that impact is associated with a wide range of other changes in the social and economic positions of women, some health-promoting and others putatively health-threatening. And since 1980 we have probably begun to gradually realize the health gains from the reductions in smoking that began in the 1960s and have continued through the present. Similarly, obesity began to spread only around 1980; its effects, especially on life expectancy, are still developing and contested. Another major social change in the United States since 1980 has been increasing immigration; immigrants, however, generally manifest higher levels of health than the native-born population, though this immigrant health advantage declines as they spend more time and generations in the United States. Trends for African Americans were variable over the latter decades of the twentieth century, sometimes improving relative to the rest of the population and sometimes worsening. Thus, America's growing racial-ethnic diversity cannot be a major explanation for our population health problems over the last several decades. In sum, none of the potential alternative explanations for America's worsening post-1980 population health problems seem more plausible than the one presented here focused on socioeconomic policy.

6. See Kingdon (1984/2011) for details on these issues. Given his formulation, Kingdon sees major policy changes as functions of major discrete policy events that occur during opportune "policy windows," rather than the result of continuing, frequent, small incremental change, necessary and useful as that kind of change also is in the total policy process. Supply-side health care and insurance policy and reforms have certainly been formulated and enacted during a number of large and widely spread "lumps" of time connected by long periods of incremental change. The same is likely to be true for the implementation of demand-side health policy, with the first major "lump" of change hopefully coming sooner rather than later.
7. It is also important to note that our current problems in health and broader social policy have developed over a period of at least four decades, during which time political power at the national and state levels in both the executive and legislative branches has been broadly shared by Republicans and Democrats. Thus, neither the origins, nature, nor potential solutions to these problems are, in my view, partisan in nature. The proposed solutions do presume, however, that all political actors care about the well-being of the broader polity and society and its major components, in addition to their own individual well-being and that of those close or similar to themselves.
8. As one example, the Robert Wood Johnson Foundation Commission to Build a Healthier America premised its work on much the same kind of evidence on declining levels of population health and growing socioeconomic and racial-ethnic disparities in health. But the commission then drew back from the logical implications of this evidence for broad socioeconomic and civil rights policy to focus on health behaviors, early childhood education, and neighborhoods and communities as arenas for presumably more politically palatable policy intervention (Robert Wood Johnson Foundation 2009).

References

Acevedo-Garcia, Dolores, Kimberly A. Lochner, Theresa L. Osypuk, and S. V. Subramanian. 2003. "Future Directions in Residential Segregation and Health Research: A Multilevel Approach." *American Journal of Public Health* 93(2): 215–21.

Acheson, Donald, David Barker, Jacky Chamber, Hilary Graham, Michael Marmot, and Margaret Whitehead. 1998. "Report of the Independent Inquiry into Inequalities in Health (Acheson Report)." London: The Stationery Office.

Ailshire, Jennifer A., and James S. House. 2011. "The Unequal Burden of Weight Gain: An Intersectional Approach to Understanding Social Disparities in BMI Trajectories from 1986 to 2001/2002." *Social Forces* 90(2): 397–423.

Almond, Douglas, Kenneth Y. Chay, and Michael Greenstone. 2006. "Civil Rights, the War on Poverty, and Black-White Convergence in Infant Mortality in the Rural South and Mississippi." Department of Economics Working Paper 07-04. Cambridge, Mass.: Massachusetts Institute of Technology.

Almond, Douglas, Hilary W. Hoynes, and Diane Whitmore Schanzenbach. 2011. "Inside the War on Poverty: The Impact of Food Stamps on Birth Outcomes." *Review of Economics and Statistics* 93(2): 387–403.

Alston, Julian M., Abigail M. Okrent, and Joanna C. Parks. 2012. "U.S. Food Policy and Obesity." In *Public Health: Social and Behavioral Health,* edited by Jay Maddock. Rijecka, Croatia: Intech. Available at: www.intechopen.com/books/public-health-social-and-behavioral-health/food-policy-and-obesity (accessed February 26, 2015).

Alston, Julian M., Daniel A. Sumner, and Stephen A. Vosti. 2008. "Farm Subsidies and Obesity in the United States: National Evidence and International Comparisons." *Food Policy* 33(6): 470–79.

American Public Health Association (APHA). 2007. "At the Intersection of Public Health and Transportation: Promoting Health Transportation Policy." Washington, D.C.: American Public Health Association.

Anderson, Wayne L., Brian S. Armour, Eric A. Finkelstein, and Joshua M. Wiener. 2010. "Estimates of State-Level Health-Care Expenditures Associated with Disability." *Public Health Reports* 125(1): 44–51.

Arno, Peter S., James S. House, Deborah Viola, and Clyde Schechter. 2011. "Social Security and Mortality: The Role of Income Support Policies and Population Health in the United States." *Journal of Public Health Policy* 32(2): 234–50.

Aronowitz, Robert A. 1998. *Making Sense of Illness: Science, Society, and Disease.* New York: Cambridge University Press.

Association of American Medical Colleges (AAMC). 2012. "MCAT 2015: A Better Test for Tomorrow's Doctors." In *Preview Guide for the MCAT 2015 Exam.* 2nd ed. Washington, D.C.: Association of American Medical Colleges.

Baicker, Katherine, Sarah L. Taubman, Heidi L. Allen, Mira Bernstein, Jonathan H. Gruber, Joseph P. Newhouse, Eric C. Schneider, Bill J. Wright, Alan M. Zaslavsky, and Amy N. Finkelstein. 2013. "The Oregon Experiment: Effects of Medicaid on Clinical Outcomes." *New England Journal of Medicine* 368(18): 1713–22.

Banthin, Jessica, and Sarah Masi. 2013. "CBO's Estimate of the Net Budgetary Impact of the Affordable Care Act's Health Insurance Coverage Provisions Has Not Changed Much over Time." CBO Blog. Washington: U.S. Government Budget Office.

Bengtsson, Tommy. 2001. "Mortality: The Great Historical Decline." In *International Encyclopedia of the Social and Behavioral Sciences,* edited by Neil J. Smelser and Paul B. Baltes. Oxford: Elsevier.

Bengtsson, Tommy, and Martin Dribe. 2011. "The Late Emergence of Socioeconomic Mortality Differentials: A Micro-Level Study of Adult Mortality in Southern Sweden, 1815–1968." *Explorations in Economic History* 48(3): 389–400.

Berkman, Lisa F., and Ichiro Kawachi. 2000. *Social Epidemiology.* New York: Oxford University Press.

Berwick, Donald M., Thomas W. Nolan, and John Whittington. 2008. "The Triple Aim: Care, Health, and Cost." *HealthAffairs* 27(3): 759–69.

Bhattacharya, Jay, and Neeraj Sood. 2011. "Who Pays for Obesity?" *Journal of Economic Perspectives* 25(1): 139–58.

Black, Ashly D., Josip Car, Claudia Pagliari, Chantelle Anandan, Kathrin Cresswell, Tomislav Bokun, Brian McKinstry, Rob Procter, Azeem Majeed, and Aziz Sheikh. 2011. "The Impact of eHealth on the Quality and Safety of Health Care: A Systematic Overview." *PLoS Medicine* 8(1): e1000387.

Black, Douglas, Jeremy N. Morris, Cyril Smith, and Peter Townsend. 1982. *Inequalities in Health: The Black Report.* New York: Penguin.

Bloom, Samuel W. 1990. "Episodes in the Institutionalization of Medical Sociology: A Personal View." *Journal of Health and Social Behavior* 31(1): 1–10.

———. 2002. *The Word as Scalpel: A History of Medical Sociology.* New York: Oxford University Press.

Blumenthal, David. 2013. "A Strong Foundation for Improving U.S. Health Care." The Commonwealth Fund, January 3. Available at: http://www.commonwealthfund.org/publications/blog/2013/jan/strong-foundation (accessed February 23, 2015).

Boardman, Jason D., Jonathan Daw, and Jeremy Freese. 2013. "Defining the Environment in Gene-Environment Research: Lessons from Social Epidemiology." *American Journal of Public Health* 103(S1): S64–72.

Bradford Hill, Austin. 1965. "The Environment and Disease: Association or Causation?" *Proceedings of the Royal Society of Medicine* 58(5): 295–300.

Bradley, Elizabeth H., Benjamin R. Elkins, Jeph Herrin, and Brian Elbel. 2011. "Health and Social Services Expenditures: Associations with Health Outcomes." *BMJ Quality and Safety* 20(10): 826–31.

Bradley, Elizabeth H., and Lauren A. Taylor. 2013. *The American Health Care Paradox: Why Spending More Is Getting Us Less.* New York: Public Affairs.

Brandt, Allan M. 2007. *The Cigarette Century: The Rise, Fall, and Deadly Persistence of the Product That Defined America.* New York: Basic Books.

Brook, Robert H., Emmett B. Keeler, Kathleen N. Lohr, Joseph P. Newhouse, John E. Ware, William H. Rogers, Allyson Ross Davies, Cathy D. Sherbourne, George A. Goldberg, Patricia Camp, Caren Kamberg, Arleen Leibowitz, Joan Keesey, and David Reboussin. 2006. "The Health Insurance Experiment: A Classic RAND Study Speaks to the Current Health Care Reform Debate." In *Research Briefs.* Santa Monica, Calif.: RAND Corporation.

Brown, Dustin C., Mark D. Hayward, Jennifer Karas Montez, Robert A. Hummer, Chi-Tsun Chiu, and Mira M. Hidajat. 2012. "The Significance of Education for Mortality Compression in the United States." *Demography* 49(3): 819–40.

Brown, L. Jackson, Thomas P. Wall, and Vickie Lazar. 2000. "Trends in Total Caries Experience: Permanent and Primary Teeth." *Journal of the American Dental Association* 131(2): 223–31.

Bunker, John P., Howard S. Frazier, and Frederick Mosteller. 1994. "Improving Health: Measuring Effects of Medical Care." *Milbank Quarterly* 72(2): 225–58.

Case, Anne. 2004. "Does Money Protect Health Status? Evidence from South African Pensions." In *Perspectives on the Economics of Aging,* edited by David A. Wise. Chicago: University of Chicago Press.

Cassel, John. 1976. "The Contribution of the Social Environment to Host Resistance." *American Journal of Epidemiology* 104(2): 107–23.

Center for Public Program Evaluation. 2011. "Surgeon General's Reports on Tobacco." RWJF Retrospective Series. Princeton, N.J.: Robert Wood Johnson Foundation.

Centers for Disease Control and Prevention. 2010. "Pregnancy Mortality Surveillance System," available at http://www.cdc.gov/reproductivehealth/MaternalInfantHealth/PMSS.html (accessed March 2, 2015).

———. 2015. "Smoking and Tobacco Use Consumption Data," available at http://web.archive.org/web/20120602155324/http://www.cdc.gov/tobacco/data_statistics/tables/economics/consumption (accessed March 2, 2015).

Centers for Medicare and Medicaid Services, Office of the Actuary. Various years. "Table 01. National Health Expenditures and Selected Indicators," available at http://www.cms.gov/Research-Statistics-Data-and-systems/Statistics-Trends-and-reports/NationalHealthExpendData/Downloads/Proj2013tables.zip (accessed February 27, 2015).

Chaudhry, Basit, Jerome Wang, Shinyi Wu, Margaret Maglione, Walter Mojica, Elizabeth Roth, Sally C. Morton, and Paul G. Shekelle. 2006. "Systematic Review: Impact of Health Information Technology on Quality, Efficiency, and Costs of Medical Care." *Annals of Internal Medicine* 144(10): 742–52.

Cheung, Siu Lan Karen, Jean-Marie Robine, Edward Jow-Ching Tu, and Graziella Caselli. 2005. "Three Dimensions of the Survival Curve: Horizontalization, Verticalization, and Longevity Extension." *Demography* 42(2): 243–58.

Cho, Youngtae, W. Parker Frisbie, Robert A. Hummer, and Richard G. Rogers. 2004. "Nativity, Duration of Residence, and the Health of Hispanic Adults in the United States." *International Migration Review* 38(1): 184–211.

Chokshi, Dave A., and Thomas A. Farley. 2012. "The Cost-Effectiveness of Environmental Approaches to Disease Prevention." *New England Journal of Medicine* 367(4): 295–97.

Clark, Rodney, Norman B. Anderson, Vernessa R. Clark, and David R. Williams. 1999. "Racism as a Stressor for African Americans: A Biopsychosocial Model." *American Psychologist* 54(10): 805–16.

Coale, Ansley. 1974. "The History of the Human Population." *Scientific American* 231(3): 41–51.

Colgrove, James. 2002. "The McKeown Thesis: A Historical Controversy and Its Enduring Influence." *American Journal of Public Health* 92(5): 725–29.

Collins, Francis S. 2004. "What We Do and Don't Know About 'Race,' 'Ethnicity,' Genetics, and Health at the Dawn of the Genome Era." *Nature Genetics* 36(11): S13–15.

Comfort, Alex. 1956. *The Biology of Senescence.* New York: Rinehart & Co.

———. 1964. *Ageing: The Biology of Senescence.* London: Routledge & Kegan Paul.

Commonwealth Fund Commission on a High Performance Health System. 2013. *Confronting Costs: Stabilizing U.S. Health Spending While Moving Toward a High Performance Health Care System.* New York: Commonwealth Fund.

Courtmanche, Charles J., and Daniela Zapata. 2014. "Does Universal Coverage Improve Health? The Massachusetts Experience." *Journal of Policy Analysis and Management* 33(1): 36–69.

Currie, Janet, and Jonathan Gruber. 1996a. "Health Insurance Eligibility, Utilization of Medical Care, and Child Health." *Quarterly Journal of Economics* 111(2): 431–66.

———. 1996b. "Saving Babies: The Efficacy and Cost of Recent Changes in the Medicaid Eligibility of Pregnant Women." *Journal of Political Economy* 104(6): 1263–96.

Cutler, David M. 2004. *Your Money or Your Life: Strong Medicine for America's Health Care System.* New York: Oxford University Press.

———. 2014. *The Quality Cure: How Focusing on Health Care Quality Can Save Your Life and Lower Spending Too.* Berkeley: University of California Press.

Cutler, David, Edward Glaeser, and Jesse Shapiro. 2003. "Why Have Americans Become More Obese?" Cambridge, Mass.: National Bureau of Economic Research.

Cutler, David M., and Adriana Lleras-Muney. 2008. "Education and Health: Evaluating Theories and Evidence." In *Making Americans Healthier: Social and Economic Policy as Health Policy,* edited by Robert F. Schoeni, James S. House, George A. Kaplan, and Harold Pollack. New York: Russell Sage Foundation.

Cutler, David M., Allison B. Rosen, and Sandeep Vijan. 2006. "The Value of Medical Spending in the United States, 1960–2000." *New England Journal of Medicine* 355(9): 920–27.

Cutler, David M., and Nikhil R. Sahni. 2013. "If Slow Rate of Health Care Spending Growth Persists, Projections May Be Off by $770 Billion." *Health Affairs* 32(5): 841–50.

Dawber, Thomas Royle. 1980. *The Framingham Study: The Epidemiology of Atherosclerotic Disease.* Cambridge, Mass.: Harvard University Press.

Dow, William H., and David H. Rehkopf. 2010. "Socioeconomic Gradients in

Health in International and Historical Context." *Annals of the New York Academy of Sciences* 1186(1): 24–36.

Dranove, David, Craig Garthwaite, and Christopher Ody. 2014. "Health Spending Slowdown Is Mostly Due to Economic Factors, Not Structural Change in the Health Care Sector." *Health Affairs* 33(8): 1399–406.

Dynarski, Susan. 2003. "Does Aid Matter? Measuring the Effect of Student Aid on College Attendance and Completion." *American Economic Review* 93(1): 279–88.

Economou, Athina, Agelike Nikolaou, and Ioannis Theodossiou. 2008. "Socioeconomic Status and Health-Care Utilization: A Study of the Effects of Low Income, Unemployment, and Hours of Work on the Demand for Health Care in the European Union." *Health Services Management Research* 21(1): 40–59.

Esping-Andersen, Gøsta. 1990. *The Three Worlds of Welfare Capitalism*. Cambridge: Polity Press.

Evans, Robert. G., and Greg L. Stoddart. 1994. "Producing Health, Consuming Health Care." In *Why Are Some People Healthy and Some Not? The Determinants of Health of Populations,* edited by Robert G. Evans, Morris L. Barer, and Theodore R. Marmor. Hawthorne, N.Y.: Aldine de Gruyter.

Evans, William N., and Craig L. Garthwaite. 2014. "Giving Mom a Break: The Impact of Higher EITC Payments on Maternal Health." *American Economic Journal: Economic Policy* 6(2): 258–90.

Fauth, Rebecca C., and Jeanne Brooks-Gunn. 2008. "Are Some Neighborhoods Better for Child Health Than Others?" In *Making Americans Healthier: Social and Economic Policy as Health Policy,* edited by Robert F. Schoeni, James S. House, George A. Kaplan, and Harold Pollack. New York: Russell Sage Foundation.

Fee, Elizabeth. 1993. "Public Health Past and Present: A Shared Social Vision." In *A History of Public Health,* expanded edition, edited by George Rosen. Baltimore: Johns Hopkins University Press.

Fernald, Lia C. H., Paul J. Gertler, and Lynnette M. Neufeld. 2008. "Role of Cash in Conditional Cash Transfer Programmes for Child Health, Growth, and Development: An Analysis of Mexico's Oportunidades." *The Lancet* 371(9615): 828–37.

Fine, Michael J., Said A. Ibrahim, and Stephen B. Thomas. 2005. "The Role of Race and Genetics in Health Disparities Research." *American Journal of Public Health* 95(12): 2125–28.

Fischer, Claude S., and Michael Hout. 2006. *Century of Difference: How America Changed in the Last One Hundred Years*. New York: Russell Sage Foundation.

Flexner, Abraham. 1910. *Medical Education in the United States and Canada*. New York: Carnegie Foundation for the Advancement of Teaching.

Fogel, Robert William. 2004. *The Escape from Hunger and Premature Death*. Cambridge: Cambridge University Press.

———. 2012. *Explaining Long-Term Trends in Health and Longevity*. New York: Cambridge University Press.

Fogel, Robert William, Roderick Floud, Bernard Harris, and Sok Chul Hong. 2011. *The Changing Body: Health, Nutrition, and Human Development in the Western World Since 1700*. New York: Cambridge University Press.

Ford, Earl S., and Simon Capewell. 2011. "Proportion of the Decline in Cardiovascular Mortality Disease Due to Prevention Versus Treatment: Public Health Versus Clinical Care." *Annual Review of Public Health* 32:5–22.

Franck, Caroline, Sonia M. Grandi, and Mark J. Eisenberg. 2013. "Agricultural Subsidies and the American Obesity Epidemic." *American Journal of Preventive Medicine* 45(3): 327–33.

Freedman, Vicki A., Eileen M. Crimmins, Robert F. Schoeni, Brenda C. Spillman, Hakan Aykan, Ellen Kramarow, Kenneth Land, James Lubitz, Kenneth Manton, Linda G. Martin, Diane Shinberg, and Timothy Waidmann. 2004. "Resolving Inconsistences in Trends in Old-Age Disability: Report from a Technical Working Group." *Demography* 41(3): 417–41.

Freeman, Howard E., Sol Levine, and Leo G. Reeder, eds. 1972. *Handbook of Medical Sociology*, 2nd ed. Englewood Cliffs, N.J.: Prentice-Hall.

Fries, James F. 1980. "Aging, Natural Death, and the Compression of Morbidity." *New England Journal of Medicine* 330(3): 130–35.

———. 2000. "Compression of Morbidity in the Elderly." *Vaccine* 18(16): 1584–89.

Fries, James F., and Lawrence M. Crapo. 1981. *Vitality and Aging*. San Francisco: W. H. Freeman.

Frost, Wade Hampton. 1936. *Introduction to Snow on Cholera*. New York: Commonwealth Fund.

Fuchs, Victor R., and Arnold Milstein. 2011. "The $640 Billion Question—Why Does Cost-Effective Care Diffuse So Slowly?" *New England Journal of Medicine* 364(21): 1985–87.

Geronimus, Arline T. 1991. "The Weathering Hypothesis and the Health of African-American Women and Infants: Evidence and Speculations." *Ethnicity and Disease* 2(3): 207–21.

———. 2001. "Understanding and Eliminating Racial Inequalities in Women's Health in the United States: The Role of the Weathering Conceptual Framework." *Journal of the American Medical Women's Association* 56(4): 133–36.

Geronimus, Arline T., John Bound, Timothy A. Waidmann, Cynthia G. Colen, and Dianne Steffick. 2001. "Inequality in Life Expectancy, Functional Status, and Active Life Expectancy Across Selected Black and White Populations in the United States." *Demography* 38(2): 227–51.

Geronimus, Arline T., Margaret T. Hicken, Danya Keene, and John Bound. 2006. "'Weathering' and Age Patterns of Allostatic Load Scores Among Blacks and Whites in the United States." *American Journal of Public Health* 96(5): 826–33.

Geronimus, Arline T., Margaret T. Hicken, Jay A. Pearson, Sarah J. Seashols, Kelly L. Brown, and Tracey Dawson Cruz. 2010. "Do U.S. Black Women Experience Stress-Related Accelerated Biological Aging?" *Human Nature* 21(1): 19–38.

Gerontologica Perspecta. 1987. Issue on "The Compression of Mortality," 1: 3–66.

Gillum, Leslie A., Christopher Gouveia, E. Ray Dorsey, Mark Pletcher, Colin D. Mathers, Charles E. McCulloch, and S. Claiborne Johnston. 2011. "NIH Disease Funding Levels and Burden of Disease." *PLoS ONE* 6(2).

Golberstein, Ezra, Richard A. Hirth, and Paula M. Lantz. 2012. "Estimating the Education-Health Relationship: A Cost-Utility Approach." *B.E. Journal of Economic Analysis and Policy* 11, issue 3 (Topics), article 7.

Goldin, Claudia Dale, and Lawrence F. Katz. 2008. *The Race Between Education and Technology*. Cambridge, Mass.: Harvard University Press.

Goldman, Lee, and E. Francis Cook. 1984. "The Decline in Ischemic Heart Disease: An Analysis of the Comparative Effects of Medical Interventions and Changes in Lifestyle." *Annals of Internal Medicine* 101(6): 825–36.

Grossman, Michael. 2000. "The Human Capital Model." In *Handbook of Health Economics,* edited by Anthony J. Cuyler and Joseph P. Newhouse. New York: Elsevier.

Hacker, Jacob S. 2002. *The Divided Welfare State: The Battle over Public and Private Social Benefits in the United States.* Cambridge: Cambridge University Press.

Haeder, Simon F. 2012. "Beyond Path Dependence: Explaining Healthcare Reform and Its Consequences." *Policy Studies Journal* 40(S1): 65–86.

Harrington, Michael. 1962. *The Other America: Poverty in the United States.* New York: Macmillan.

Hartman, Micah, Anne B. Martin, Joseph Benson, and Aaron Catlin. 2013. "National Health Spending in 2011: Overall Growth Remains Low, but Some Payers and Services Show Signs of Acceleration." *Health Affairs* 32(1): 87–99.

Hauser, Philip M. 1953. "Facing the Implications of an Aging Population." *Social Service Review* 27:162–76.

Herd, Pamela, Brian Goesling, and James S. House. 2007. "Socioeconomic Position and Health: The Differential Effects of Education *versus* Income on the Onset *versus* Progression of Health Problems." *Journal of Health and Social Behavior* 48(3): 223–38.

Herd, Pamela, James S. House, and Robert F. Schoeni. 2008. "Income Support Policies and Health Among the Elderly." In *Making Americans Healthier: Social and Economic Policy as Health Policy,* edited by Robert F. Schoeni, James S. House, George A. Kaplan, and Harold Pollack. New York: Russell Sage Foundation.

Herd, Pamela, Robert F. Schoeni, and James S. House. 2008. "Upstream Solutions: Does the Supplemental Security Income Program Reduce Disability in the Elderly?" *Milbank Quarterly* 86(1): 5–45.

Hicken, Margaret T., Hedwig Lee, Jeffrey Morenoff, James S. House, and David R. Williams. 2014. "Racial/Ethnic Disparities in Hypertension Prevalence: Reconsidering the Role of Chronic Stress." *American Journal of Public Health* 104(1): 117–23.

Hirth, Richard A., Michael E. Chernew, Edward Miller, A. Mark Fendrick, and William G. Weissert. 2000. "Willingness to Pay for a Quality-Adjusted Life Year: In Search of a Standard." *Medical Decision Making* 20(3): 332–42.

Ho, Jessica Y., and Samuel H. Preston. 2010. "U.S. Mortality in an International Context: Age Variations." *Population and Development Review* 36(4): 749–73.

House, James S. 2002. "Understanding Social Factors and Inequalities in Health: 20th Century Progress and 21st Century Prospects." *Journal of Health and Social Behavior* 43:125–42.

House, James S., Karl R. Landis, and Debra Umberson. 1988. "Social Relationships and Health." *Science* 241:540–45.

House, James S., Ronald C. Kessler, Anna Regula Herzog, Richard Mero, Ann Kinney, and Martha Breslow. 1990. "Age, Socioeconomic Status, and Health." *Milbank Quarterly* 68(3): 383–411.

House, James S., Paula M. Lantz, and Pamela Herd. 2005. "Continuity and Change in the Social Stratification of Aging and Health over the Life Course:

Evidence from a Nationally Representative Longitudinal Study from 1986 to 2001–2002 (Americans' Changing Lives Study)." *Journals of Gerontology: Series B* 60B (Special Issue II):15–26.

House, James S., James M. Lepkowski, Ann M. Kinney, Richard P. Mero, Ronald C. Kessler, and Anna Regula Herzog. 1994. "The Social Stratification of Aging and Health." *Journal of Health and Social Behavior* 35(3): 213–34.

House, James S., and David R. Williams. 2000. "Understanding and Reducing Socioeconomic and Racial/Ethnic Disparities in Health." In *Promoting Health: Intervention Strategies from Social and Behavioral Research*, edited by Brian D. Smedley and Leonard S. Syme. Washington, D.C.: National Academies Press.

Hoynes, Hilary W., Douglas L. Miller, and David Simon. 2012. "Income, the Earned Income Tax Credit, and Infant Health." Cambridge, Mass.: National Bureau of Economic Research.

Hummer, Robert A., and Juanita J. Chinn. 2011. "Race/Ethnicity and U.S. Adult Mortality." *Du Bois Review* 8(1): 5–24.

Hummer, Robert A., and Elaine M. Hernandez. 2013. "The Effect of Educational Attainment on Adult Mortality in the United States." *Population Bulletin* 68(1): 1–18.

Hummer, Robert A., Jennifer E. Melvin, Connor M. Sheehan, and Ying-Ting Wang. 2013. "Race/Ethnicity, Mortality, and Longevity." In *The Handbook of Minority Aging*, edited by Keith E. Whitfield and Tamara A. Baker. New York: Springer Publishing Co.

Hummer, Robert A., Richard G. Rogers, Charles B. Nam, and Christopher G. Ellison. 1999a. "Religious Involvement and U.S. Adult Mortality." *Demography* 36(2): 273–85.

Hummer, Robert A., Richard G. Rogers, Charles B. Nam, and Felicia B. LeClere. 1999b. "Race/Ethnicity, Nativity, and U.S. Adult Mortality." *Social Science Quarterly* 80(1): 136–53.

Hunink, Maria G. M., Lee Goldman, Anna N. A. Tosteson, Murray A. Mittleman, Paula A. Goldman, Lawrence W. Williams, Joel Tsevat, and Milton C. Weinstein. 1997. "The Recent Decline in Mortality from Coronary Heart Disease, 1980–1990." *Journal of the American Medical Association* 277(7): 535–42.

Johnson, Rucker C. 2011. "Long-Run Impacts of School Desegregation and School Quality on Adult Attainments." Cambridge, Mass.: National Bureau of Economic Research.

Kahneman, Daniel. 2011. *Thinking, Fast and Slow.* New York: Farrar, Straus, and Giroux.

Kaplan, George A., Nalini Ranjit, and Sarah A. Burgard. 2008. "Lifting Gates, Lengthening Lives: Did Civil Rights Policies Improve the Health of African American Women in the 1960s and 1970s?" In *Making Americans Healthier: Social and Economic Policy as Health Policy*, edited by Robert F. Schoeni, James S. House, George A. Kaplan, and Harold Pollack. New York: Russell Sage Foundation.

Kawachi, Ichiro, and Lisa F. Berkman, eds. 2003. *Neighborhoods and Health.* New York: Oxford University Press.

Keating, Daniel P., and Sharon Z. Simonton. 2008. "Health Effects of Human Development Policies." In *Making Americans Healthier: Social and Economic Policy as Health Policy,* edited by Robert F. Schoeni, James S. House, George A. Kaplan, and Harold Pollack. New York: Russell Sage Foundation.

Kellermann, Arthur L., and Spencer S. Jones. 2013. "What It Will Take to Achieve the As-Yet-Unfulfilled Promises of Health Information Technology." *Health Affairs* 32(1): 63–68.

Keskimäki, Ilmo, Marjo Salinto, and Seppo Aro. 1995. "Socioeconomic Equity in Finnish Hospital Care in Relation to Need." *Social Science and Medicine* 41(3): 425–31.

Kessler, Ronald C., J. Blake Turner, and James S. House. 1988. "Effects of Unemployment on Health in a Community Survey: Main, Modifying, and Mediating Effects." *Journal of Social Issues* 44(4): 69–85.

Keynes, John Maynard. 1923. *A Tract on Monetary Reform.* London: Macmillan.

Kindig, David A., and Erika R. Cheng. 2013. "Even as Mortality Fell in Most U.S. Counties, Female Mortality Nonetheless Rose in 42.8 Percent of Counties from 1992 to 2006." *Health Affairs* 32(3): 451–58.

Kindig, David, and John Mullahy. 2010. "Comparative Effectiveness—of What? Evaluating Strategies to Improve Population Health." *Journal of the American Medical Association* 304(8): 901–2.

Kingdon, John W. 2011. *Agendas, Alternatives, and Public Policies.* Updated 2nd edition with epilogue. Upper Saddle River, N.J.: Pearson. (Originally published in 1984.)

Kling, Jeffrey R., Jeffrey B. Liebman, and Lawrence F. Katz. 2007. "Experimental Analysis of Neighborhood Effects." *Econometrica* 75(1): 83–119.

Kluger, Richard. 1997. *Ashes to Ashes: America's Hundred-Year Cigarette War, the Public Health, and the Unabashed Triumph of Philip Morris.* New York: Vintage.

Kochanek, Kenneth D., Jiaquan Xu, Sherry L. Murphy, Arialdi M. Miniño, and Hsiang-Ching Kung. "Deaths: Preliminary Data for 2009." *National Vital Statistics Report* 59(4, March 16). Available at: http://www.cdc.gov/nchs/data/nvsr/nvsr59/nvsr59_04.pdf (accessed February 23, 2015).

Kulkarni, Sandeep C., Alison Levin-Rector, Majid Ezzati, and Christopher J. L. Murray. 2011. "Falling Behind: Life Expectancy in U.S. Counties from 2000 to 2007 in an International Context." *Population Health Metrics* 9(1): 16.

Lantz, Paula M., Ezra Golberstein, James S. House, and Jeffrey Morenoff. 2010. "Socioeconomic and Behavioral Risk Factors for Mortality in a National 19-Year Prospective Study of U.S. Adults." *Social Science and Medicine* 70(10): 1558–66.

Lantz, Paula M., James S. House, James M. Lepkowski, David R. Williams, Richard P. Mero, and Jieming Chen. 1998. "Socioeconomic Factors, Health Behaviors, and Mortality: Results from a Nationally Representative Prospective Study of U.S. Adults." *Journal of the American Medical Association* 279(21): 1703–8.

Lantz, Paula M., James S. House, Richard P. Mero, and David R. Williams. 2005. "Stress, Life Events, and Socioeconomic Disparities in Health: Results from the Americans' Changing Lives Study." *Journal of Health and Social Behavior* 46(3): 274–88.

LaVeist, Thomas A. 2005. *Minority Populations and Health: An Introduction to Health Disparities in the United States.* San Francisco: Jossey-Bass.

Levy, Helen, and David Meltzer. 2001. "What Do We Really Know About Whether Health Insurance Affects Health?" In *Health Policy and the Uninsured*, edited by Catherine G. McLaughlin. Washington, D.C.: Urban Institute Press.

———. 2008. "The Impact of Health Insurance on Health." *Annual Review of Public Health* 29:399–409.

Levy, Michel Louis. 1996. "La Rectangularisation de la courbe des survivants" ("The Rectangularization of the Survival Curve"). In *Morbidité, mortalité: Problemes de mesure, facteurs d'evolution, essai de prospective: Colloque international de Sinaia (2–6 Septembre 1996)* (*Morbidity, Mortality: Problems of Measurement, Factors of Evolution, Prospective Trials: International Symposium in Sinaia, September 2–6, 1996*), edited by Association Internationale des Démographes de Langue Française. Paris: Presses Universitaires de France.

Link, Bruce G., and Jo C. Phelan. 1995. "Social Conditions as Fundamental Causes of Disease." *Journal of Health and Social Behavior* (extra issue):80–94.

———. 2000. "Evaluating the Fundamental Cause Explanation for Social Disparities in Health." In *Handbook of Medical Sociology*, 5th ed., edited by Chloe E. Bird, Peter Conrad, and Allen Fremont. Upper Saddle River, N.J.: Prentice-Hall.

Ludwig, Jens, Lisa Sanbonmatsu, Lisa Gennetian, Emma Adam, Greg J. Duncan, Lawrence F. Katz, Ronald C. Kessler, Jeffrey R. Kling, Stacy Tessler Lindau, and Robert C. Whitaker. 2011. "Neighborhoods, Obesity, and Diabetes: A Randomized Social Experiment." *New England Journal of Medicine* 365(16): 1509–19.

Lynch, John W., George A. Kaplan, Richard D. Cohen, Jaakko Tuomilehto, and Jukka T. Salonen. 1996. "Do Cardiovascular Risk Factors Explain the Relation Between Socioeconomic Status, Risk of All-Cause Mortality, Cardiovascular Mortality, and Acute Myocardial Infarction?" *American Journal of Epidemiology* 144(10): 934–42.

Mackenbach, Johan P. 2011. "Can We Reduce Health Inequalities? An Analysis of the English Strategy (1997–2010)." *Journal of Epidemiology and Community Health* 65(7): 568–75.

Manton, Kenneth G., and H. Dennis Tolley. 1991. "Rectangularization of the Survival Curve: Implications of an Ill-Posed Question." *Journal of Aging and Health* 3(2): 172–93.

Marmot, Michael G., Manolis Kogevinas, and Mary Ann Elston. 1987. "Social/Economic Status and Disease." *Annual Review of Public Health* 8:111–35.

Martel, Sylvie, and Robert Bourbeau. 2003. "Compression de la mortalité et rectangularisation de la courbe de survie au Québec au cours du XXe Siècle" ("Compression of Mortality and Rectangularization of the Survival Curve in Quebec in the Twentieth Century"), *Cahiers Québéçois de Démographie* 32(1): 43–75.

Martin, Linda G., and Robert F. Schoeni. 2014. "Trends in Disability and Related Chronic Conditions Among the Forty-and-Over Population." *Disability and Health Journal* 7(1): S4–14.

Massey, Douglas S., and Nancy A. Denton. 1993. *American Apartheid: Segregation and the Making of the Underclass.* Cambridge, Mass.: Harvard University Press.

Matthews, Karen A., Linda C. Gallo, and Shelley E. Taylor. 2010. "Are Psychosocial Factors Mediators of Socioeconomic Status and Health Connections?" *Annals of the New York Academy of Sciences* 1186(1): 146–73.

McGinnis, J. Michael, Pamela Williams-Russo, and James R. Knickman. 2002. "The Case for More Active Policy Attention to Health Promotion." *Health Affairs* 21(2): 78–93.

McGuire, Thomas G., and Jeanne Miranda. 2008. "New Evidence Regarding Racial and Ethnic Disparities in Mental Health: Policy Implications." *Health Affairs* 27(2): 393–403.

McKeown, Thomas. 1976. *The Modern Rise of Population.* London: Edward Arnold.

———. 1979. *The Role of Medicine: Dream, Mirage, or Nemesis?* Princeton, N.J.: Princeton University Press.

———. 1988. *The Origins of Human Disease.* London: Blackwell.

McKeown, Thomas, and Reginald G. Record. 1962. "Reasons for the Decline of Mortality in England and Wales During the Nineteenth Century." *Population Studies* 16(2): 94–122.

McKinlay, John B., and Sonja J. McKinlay. 1977. "The Questionable Contribution of Medical Measures to the Decline of Mortality in the United States in the Twentieth Century." *Milbank Memorial Fund Quarterly* 55(3): 405–28.

Mehta, Neil, James S. House, and Michael R. Elliott, forthcoming. "Dynamics of Health Behaviors and Socioeconomic Differences in Mortality in the USA." *Journal of Epidemiology and Community Health.*

Michalopoulos, Charles, David Wittenburg, Dina A. R. Israel, and Anne Warren. 2012. "The Effects of Health Care Benefits on Health Care Use and Health: A Randomized Trial for Disability Insurance Beneficiaries." *Medical Care* 50(9): 764–71.

Michaud, Pierre-Carl, Dana Goldman, Darius Lakdawalla, Adam Gailey, and Yuhui Zheng. 2011. "Differences in Health Between Americans and Western Europeans: Effects on Longevity and Public Finance." *Social Science and Medicine* 73(2): 254–63.

Mitra, Sophie, Patricia A. Findley, and Usha Sambamoorthi. 2009. "Health Care Expenditures of Living with a Disability: Total Expenditures, Out-of-Pocket Expenses, and Burden, 1996 to 2004." *Archives of Physical Medicine and Rehabilitation* 90(9): 1532–40.

Montez, Jennifer K., Robert A. Hummer, Mark D. Hayward, Hyeyoung Woo, and Richard G. Rogers. 2011. "Trends in the Educational Gradient of U.S. Adult Mortality from 1986 Through 2006 by Race, Gender, and Age Group." *Research on Aging* 33(2): 145–71.

Montez, Jennifer K., and Anna Zajacova. 2013a. "Explaining the Widening Education Gap in Mortality Among U.S. White Women." *Journal of Health and Social Behavior* 54(2): 166–82.

———. 2013b. "Trends in Mortality Risk by Education Level and Cause of Death Among U.S. White Women from 1986 to 2006." *American Journal of Public Health* 103(3): 473–79.

Morenoff, Jeffrey D., Ana V. Diez Roux, Ben B. Hansen, and Theresa L. Osypuk. 2008. "Residential Environments and Obesity: What Can We Learn About Policy Interventions from Observational Studies?" In *Making Americans Healthier: Social and Economic Policy as Health Policy,* edited by Robert F. Schoeni, James S. House, George A. Kaplan, and Harold Pollack. New York: Russell Sage Foundation.

Morenoff, Jeffrey D., James S. House, Ben B. Hansen, David R. Williams, George A. Kaplan, and Haslyn E. R. Hunte. 2007. "Understanding Social Disparities in Hypertension Prevalence, Awareness, Treatment, and Control: The Role of Neighborhood Context." *Social Science and Medicine* 65(9): 1853–66.

Murphy, Kevin M., and Robert H. Topel. 2006. "The Value of Health and Longevity." *Journal of Political Economy* 114(5): 871–904.

Musick, Marc A., James S. House, and David R. Williams. 2004. "Attendance at Religious Services and Mortality in a National Sample." *Journal of Health and Social Behavior* 45(2): 198–213.

National Cancer Institute Surveillance, Epidemiology, and End Results (SEER) Program. Various years. "SEER Cancer Statistics Review, 1975–2007," available at: http://seer.cancer.gov/csr/1975_2007/sections.html (accessed February 19, 2015).

National Institutes of Health (NIH). Office of Budget. Various years. *Appropriations History.* Available at: http://officeofbudget.od.nih.gov/approp_hist.html (accessed February 23, 2015).

National Institutes of Health (NIH). Office of Behavioral and Social Sciences Research. 2005. "Outcome Assessment of NIH Activities in Behavioral and Social Sciences Research." March. Available at: http://obssr.od.nih.gov/about_obssr/history/BSSR_program_outcome_assessment/prog_outcome_assess.aspx (accessed February 23, 2015).

———. 2008. "Strategic Plan for Basic Behavioral Research." July. Available at: http://obssr.od.nih.gov/pdf/bBSSR%20StrategicPlanOBSSR%20FINAL.pdf (accessed February 23, 2015).

National Research Council (NRC). 2011a. *Explaining Divergent Levels of Longevity in High-Income Countries.* Washington, D.C.: National Academies Press.

———. 2011b. *Improving Health in the United States: The Role of Health Impact Assessment.* Washington, D.C.: National Academies Press.

———. 2011c. *International Differences in Mortality at Older Ages.* Washington, D.C.: National Academies Press.

National Research Council (NRC) and Institute of Medicine. 2013. *U.S. Health in International Perspective: Shorter Lives, Poorer Health.* Washington, D.C.: National Academies Press.

Newman, Katherine S. 2003. *A Different Shade of Gray: Midlife and Beyond in the Inner City.* New York: New Press.

Oberlander, Jonathan. 2011. "Long Time Coming: Why Health Reform Finally Passed." *Health Affairs* 29(6): 1112–16.

———. 2012a. "The Future of Obamacare." *New England Journal of Medicine* 367(23): 2165–67.

———. 2012b. "Unfinished Journey—A Century of Health Care Reform in the United States." *New England Journal of Medicine* 367(7): 585–90.

Okrent, Abigail M., and Julian M. Alston. 2012. "The Effects of Farm Commodity and Retail Food Policies on Obesity and Economic Welfare in the United States." *American Journal of Agricultural Economics* 94(3): 611–46.

Olshansky, S. Jay, Toni Antonucci, Lisa Berkman, Robert H. Binstock, Axel Boersch-Supan, John T. Cacioppo, Bruce A. Carnes, Laura L. Carstensen, Linda P. Fried, Dana P. Goldman, James Jackson, Martin Kohli, John Rother, Yuhui

Zheng, and John Rowe. 2012. "Differences in Life Expectancy Due to Race and Educational Differences Are Widening, and Many May Not Catch Up." *Health Affairs* 31(8): 1803–13.

Omran, Abdel R. 1971. "The Epidemiologic Transition: A Theory of the Epidemiology of Population Change." *Milbank Memorial Fund Quarterly* 49(4): 509–38.

Organization for Economic Cooperation and Development (OECD). 2009. "Health at a Glance 2009: OECD Indicators," available at http://www.sourceoecd.org/9789264061538 (accessed November 10, 2010).

———. 2010. "OECD Factbook 2010: Economic, Environmental and Social Statistics," available at http://www.oecd-ilibrary.org/social-issues-migration-health/oecd-factbook-2010/life-expectancy_factbook-2010-85-en (accessed November 4, 2010).

———. 2013a. *Education at a Glance 2013: OECD Indicators.* Paris: OECD Publishing.

———. 2013b. *OECD Factbook 2013.* Paris: OECD Publishing.

———. 2014. *Education at a Glance 2014: OECD Indicators.* Paris: OECD Publishing.

OECD iLibrary. Various years. "OECD Health Data: Health Expenditure and Financing," DOI: 10.1787/data-00349-en (accessed February 26, 2015).

OECD.StatExtracts. Various years. "Health Status," available at: http://stats.oecd.org/index.aspx?DataSetCode=HEALTH_STAT# (accessed February 18, 2015).

Pamuk, Elsie R., Diane M. Makuc, Katherine E. Heck, Cynthia Reuben, and Kimberly A. Lochner. 1998. *Socioeconomic Status and Health Chartbook. Health, United States, 1998.* Hyattsville, Md.: National Center for Health Statistics.

Pappas, Greg, Susan Queen, Wilbur Hadden, and Gail Fisher. 1993. "The Increasing Disparity in Mortality Between Socioeconomic Groups in the United States, 1960 and 1986." *New England Journal of Medicine* 329(2): 103–9.

Pascoe, Elizabeth A., and Laura Smart Richman. 2009. "Perceived Discrimination and Health: A Meta-Analytic Review." *Psychological Bulletin* 135(4): 531.

Paxson, Christina H., and Norbert Rüdiger Schady. 2007. "Does Money Matter?: The Effects of Cash Transfers on Child Health and Development in Rural Ecuador." Policy Research Working Paper 4226. Washington, D.C.: World Bank.

Pearce, Neil, Sunia Foliaki, Andrew Spole, and Chris Cunningham. 2004. "Genetics, Race, Ethnicity, and Health." *British Medical Journal* 328(7447): 1070.

Phelan, Jo C., Bruce G. Link, Ana Diez-Roux, Ichiro Kawachi, and Bruce Levin. 2004. "'Fundamental Causes' of Social Inequalities in Mortality: A Test of the Theory." *Journal of Health and Social Behavior* 45(3): 265–85.

Phelan, Jo C., Bruce G. Link, and Parisa Tehranifar. 2010. "Social Conditions as Fundamental Causes of Health Inequalities: Theory, Evidence, and Policy Implications." *Journal of Health and Social Behavior* 51(supplement 1): S28–40.

Piketty, Thomas. 2014. *Capital in the Twenty-First Century.* Cambridge, Mass.: Belknap Press of Harvard University Press.

Pollan, Michael. 2006. *The Omnivore's Dilemma: A Natural History of Four Meals.* New York: Penguin Press.

Preston, Samuel H., and Michael R. Haines. 1991. *Fatal Years: Child Mortality in Late Nineteenth-Century America.* Princeton, N.J.: Princeton University Press.

Puska, Pekka, and Timo Ståhl. 2010. "Health in All Policies: The Finnish Initiative: Background, Principles, and Current Issues." *Annual Review of Public Health* 31:315–28.

Quadagno, Jill S. 2006. *One Nation, Uninsured: Why the U.S. Has No National Health Insurance.* New York: Oxford University Press.

Raynault, Eloisa, and Ed Christopher. 2013. "How Does Transportation Affect Public Health?" *Public Roads* 76(6): 29–34.

Razzell, Peter, and Christine Spence. 2006. "The Hazards of Wealth: Adult Mortality in Pre-Twentieth-Century England." *Social History of Medicine* 19(3): 381–405.

Relman, Arnold S. 1980. "The New Medical-Industrial Complex." *New England Journal of Medicine* 303(17): 963–70.

———. 1991. "Shattuck Lecture: The Health Care Industry: Where Is It Taking Us?" *New England Journal of Medicine* 325(12): 854–59.

———. 2014. "A Challenge to American Doctors." *New York Review of Books* 61(13, August 14). Available at: http://www.nybooks.com/articles/archives/2014/aug/14/challenge-american-doctors/?insrc=toc (accessed October 8, 2014).

Rieker, Patricia P., and Chloe E. Bird. 2000. "Sociological Explanations of Gender Differences in Mental and Physical Health." In *Handbook of Medical Sociology,* 5th ed., edited by Chloe E. Bird, Peter Conrad, and Allen M. Fremont. Upper Saddle River, N.J.: Prentice-Hall.

Rieker, Patricia P., Chloe E. Bird, and Martha E. Lang. 2010. "Understanding Gender and Health: Old Patterns, New Trends, and Future Directions." In *Handbook of Medical Sociology,* 6th ed., edited by Chloe E. Bird, Peter Conrad, Allen M. Fremont, and Stefan Timmermans. Nashville, Tenn.: Vanderbilt University Press.

Riley, James C. 2001. *Rising Life Expectancy: A Global History.* New York: Cambridge University Press.

Robertson, Leon S. 1996. "Reducing Death on the Road: The Effects of Minimum Safety Standards, Publicized Crash Tests, Seat Belts, and Alcohol." *American Journal of Public Health* 86(1): 31–34.

———. 2006. "Motor Vehicle Deaths: Failed Policy Analysis and Neglected Policy." *Journal of Public Health Policy* 27(2): 182–89.

Robert Wood Johnson Foundation Commission to Build a Healthier America. 2009. *Beyond Health Care: New Directions to a Healthier America,* edited by Wilhelmine Miller, Patti Simon, and Saqi Maleque. Princeton, N.J.: Robert Wood Johnson Foundation.

Rosen, George. 1958. *A History of Public Health.* New York: MD Publications.

———. 1979. "The Evolution of Social Medicine." In *Handbook of Medical Sociology,* edited by Howard Freeman, Sol Levine, and Leo G. Reeder. Englewood Cliffs, N.J.: Prentice-Hall.

———. 1993. *A History of Public Health,* expanded edition. Baltimore: Johns Hopkins University Press.

Rosenfeld, Jake. 2014. *What Unions No Longer Do.* Cambridge, Mass.: Harvard University Press.

Ross, Catherine E., and John Mirowsky. 2000. "Does Medical Insurance Contribute to Socioeconomic Differentials in Health?" *Milbank Quarterly* 78(2): 291–321.

Rostron, Brian L., John L. Boies, and Elizabeth Arias. 2010. *Education Reporting and Classification on Death Certificates in the United States.* Washington: U.S. Department of Health and Human Services, Centers for Disease Control and Prevention, National Center for Health Statistics.

Ruhm, Christopher J. 2008. "Macroeconomic Conditions, Health, and Government Policy." In *Making Americans Healthier: Social and Economic Policy as Health Policy,* edited by Robert F. Schoeni, James S. House, George A. Kaplan, and Harold Pollack. New York: Russell Sage Foundation.

Ryu, Alexander J., Teresa B. Gibson, M. Richard McKellar, and Michael E. Chernew. 2013. "The Slowdown in Health Care Spending in 2009–11 Reflected Factors Other Than the Weak Economy and Thus May Persist." *Health Affairs* 32(5): 835–40.

Sanbonmatsu, Lisa, Lawrence F. Katz, Jens Ludwig, Lisa A. Gennetian, Greg J. Duncan, Ronald C. Kessler, Emma Adam, Thomas W. McDade, and Stacy Tessler Lindau. 2011. *Moving to Opportunity for Fair Housing Demonstration Program: Final Impacts Evaluation.* Washington: U.S. Department of Housing and Urban Development (November).

Sankar, Pamela, Mildred K. Cho, Celeste M. Condit, Linda M. Hunt, Barbara Koenig, Patricia Marshall, Sandra Soo-Jin Lee, and Paul Spicer. 2004. "Genetic Research and Health Disparities." *Journal of the American Medical Association* 291(24): 2985–89.

Schneider, Edward L., and Jacob A. Brody. 1983. "Aging, Natural Death, and the Compression of Morbidity: Another View." *New England Journal of Medicine* 309(14): 854–57.

Schoeni, Robert F., William H. Dow, Wilhelmine D. Miller, and Elsie R. Pamuk. 2011. "The Economic Value of Improving the Health of Disadvantaged Americans." *American Journal of Preventive Medicine* 40(1): S67–72.

Schoeni, Robert F., James S. House, George A. Kaplan, and Harold Pollack, eds. 2008. *Making Americans Healthier: Social and Economic Policy as Health Policy.* New York: Russell Sage Foundation.

Schoeni, Robert F., Linda G. Martin, Patricia M. Andreski, and Vicki A. Freedman. 2005. "Persistent and Growing Socioeconomic Disparities in Disability Among the Elderly: 1982–2002." *American Journal of Public Health* 95(11): 2065–70.

Silvertown, Jonathan. 2013. *The Long and the Short of It: The Science of Life Span and Aging.* Chicago: University of Chicago Press.

Sisko, Andrea M., Christopher J. Truffer, Sean P. Keehan, John A. Poisal, M. Kent Clemens, and Andrew J. Madison. 2010. "National Health Spending Projections: The Estimated Impact of Reform Through 2019." *Health Affairs* 29(10): 1933–41.

Smedley, Brian D., Adrienne Y. Stith, and Alan R. Nelson, eds. 2003. *Unequal Treatment: Confronting Racial and Ethnic Disparities in Health Care.* Washington, D.C.: National Academies Press.

Sommers, Benjamin D., Sharon K. Long, and Katherine Baicker. 2014. "Changes in Mortality After Massachusetts Health Care Reform." *Annals of Internal Medicine* 160(9): 585–94.

Ståhl, Timo, Matthias Wismar, Eeva Ollila, Eero Lahtinen, and Kimmo Leppo, eds. 2006. *Health in All Policies: Prospects and Potentials*. Helsinki: Finnish Ministry of Social Affairs and Health.

Starr, Paul. 1982. *The Social Transformation of American Medicine*. New York: Basic Books.

Strawbridge, William J., Richard D. Cohen, Sarah J. Shema, and George A. Kaplan. 1997. "Frequent Attendance at Religious Services and Mortality over 28 Years." *American Journal of Public Health* 87(6): 957–61.

Sullivan, Daniel, and Till von Wachter. 2009a. "Average Earnings and Long-Term Mortality: Evidence from Administrative Data." *American Economic Review* 99(2): 133–38.

———. 2009b. "Job Displacement and Mortality: An Analysis Using Administrative Data." *Quarterly Journal of Economics* 124(3): 1265–306.

Surgeon General's Advisory Committee on Smoking and Health. 1964. "Smoking and Health: Report of the Advisory Committee to the Surgeon General of the Public Health Service." Washington: U.S. Public Health Service, Office of the Surgeon General.

Sytkowski, Pamela A., William B. Kannel, and Ralph B. D'Agostino. 1990. "Changes in Risk Factors and the Decline in Mortality from Cardiovascular Disease: The Framingham Heart Study." *New England Journal of Medicine* 322(23): 1635–41.

Szreter, Simon. 2002. "Rethinking McKeown: The Relationship Between Public Health and Social Change." *American Journal of Public Health* 92(5): 722–25.

Tapia Granados, José A. 2005a. "Increasing Mortality During the Expansions of the U.S. Economy, 1900–1996." *International Journal of Epidemiology* 34(6): 1194–1202.

———. 2005b. "Recessions and Mortality in Spain, 1980–1997." *European Journal of Population* 21(4): 393–422.

———. 2008. "Macroeconomic Fluctuations and Mortality in Postwar Japan." *Demography* 45(2): 323–43.

Tapia Granados, José A., and Ana V. Diez Roux. 2009. "Life and Death During the Great Depression." *Proceedings of the National Academy of Sciences* 106(41): 17290–95.

Tapia Granados, José A., James S. House, Edward L. Ionides, Sarah Burgard, and Robert F. Schoeni. 2014. "Individual Joblessness, Contextual Unemployment, and Mortality Risk." *American Journal of Epidemiology* 180(2): 280–87.

Taubman, Paul, and Robin C. Sickles. 1983. "Supplemental Social Insurance and the Health of the Poor." NBER Working Paper 1062. Cambridge, Mass.: National Bureau of Economic Research.

Taylor, Shelley E., Rena L. Repetti, and Teresa Seeman. 1997. "Health Psychology: What Is an Unhealthy Environment and How Does It Get Under the Skin?" *Annual Review of Psychology* 48:411–47.

The Economists' Voice. 2010. Entire issue, 7(5).

Titmuss, Richard Morris. 1958. *Essays on "The Welfare State."* London: Allen & Unwin.

Tversky, Amos, and Daniel Kahneman. 1974. "Judgment Under Uncertainty: Heuristics and Biases." *Science* 185(4157): 1124–31.

Ubel, Peter A., Richard A. Hirth, Michael E. Chernew, and A. Mark Fendrick.

2003. "What Is the Price of Life and Why Doesn't It Increase at the Rate of Inflation?" *Archives of Internal Medicine* 163(14): 1637.

Unal, Belgin, Julia Alison Critchley, and Simon Capewell. 2004. "Explaining the Decline in Coronary Heart Disease Mortality in England and Wales Between 1981 and 2000." *Circulation* 109(9): 1101–7.

UN Demographic Yearbook. 1950. Available at http://unstats.un.org/unsd/demographic/products/dyb/dyb2.htm (accessed February 27, 2015).

U.S. Census Bureau. 2012. "Statistical Abstract of the United States: 2012," available at https://www.census.gov/compendia/statab/2012/tables/12s0117.pdf (accessed March 2, 2015).

Van der Wees, Philip J., Alan M. Zaslavsky, and John Z. Ayanian. 2013. "Improvements in Health Status After Massachusetts Health Care Reform." *Milbank Quarterly* 91(4): 663–89.

Van Poppel, Frans, Roel Jennissen, and Kees Mandemakers. 2009. "Time Trends in Social Class Mortality Differentials in the Netherlands, 1820–1920: An Assessment Based on Indirect Estimation Techniques." *Social Science History* 33(2): 119–53.

Vaupel, James W. 2010. "Biodemography of Human Ageing." *Nature* 464(7288): 536–42.

Verbrugge, Lois M. 1984. "Longer Life but Worsening Health? Trends in Health and Mortality of Middle-Aged and Older Persons." *Milbank Memorial Fund Quarterly/Health and Society* 62(3): 475–519.

Verbrugge, Lois M., and Deborah L. Wingard. 1987. "Sex Differentials in Health and Mortality." *Women and Health* 12(2): 103–45.

Wilkins, Russell, Owen Adams, and Anna Brancker. 1989. "Changes in Mortality by Income in Urban Canada from 1971 to 1986." *Health Reports* 1(2): 137–74.

Williams, David R. 1994. "The Concept of Race in Health Services Research: 1966 to 1990." *Health Services Research* 29(3): 261–74.

Williams, David R., and Chiquita Collins. 2013. "Racial Residential Segregation: A Fundamental Cause of Racial Disparities in Health." In *Race, Ethnicity, and Health: A Public Health Reader,* ed. Thomas A. LaVeist and Lydia A. Isaac. San Francisco: Jossey-Bass.

Williams, David R., Mark B. McClellan, and Alice M. Rivlin. 2010. "Beyond the Affordable Care Act: Achieving Real Improvements in Americans' Health." *Health Affairs* 29(8): 1481–88.

Williams, David R., and Selina A. Mohammed. 2009. "Discrimination and Racial Disparities in Health: Evidence and Needed Research." *Journal of Behavioral Medicine* 32(1): 20–47.

Williams, David R., Harold W. Neighbors, and James S. Jackson. 2003. "Racial/Ethnic Discrimination and Health: Findings from Community Studies." *American Journal of Public Health* 93(2): 200–208.

Wilmoth, John R., and Shiro Horiuchi. 1999. "Rectangularization Revisited: Variability of Age at Death Within Human Populations." *Demography* 36(4): 475–95.

World Health Organization. 2013. "Gender, Women, and Health: What Do We Mean by 'Sex' and 'Gender'?" Available at: http://www.who.int/gender/whatisgender/en/ (accessed September 13, 2013).

Xu, K. Tom, Brian K. Nelson, and Steven Berk. 2009. "The Changing Profile of

Patients Who Used Emergency Department Services in the United States: 1996 to 2005." *Annals of Emergency Medicine* 54(6): 805–10.

Young, T. Kue. 1998. *Population Health: Concepts and Methods.* New York: Oxford University Press.

Zimmer, Zachary, and James S. House. 2003. "Education, Income, and Functional Limitation Transitions Among American Adults: Contrasting Onset and Progression." *International Journal of Epidemiology* 32(6): 1089–97.

Index

Boldface numbers refer to figures and tables.

CPSIA information can be obtained
at www.ICGtesting.com
Printed in the USA
BVOW06s2117040118
504515BV00009B/61/P